MEASUREMENT INSTRUMENTS IN CLINICAL ETHICS

MEASUREMENT INSTRUMENTS IN CLINICAL ETHICS

BARBARA KLUG REDMAN
Wayne State University

Sage Publications
International Educational and Professional Publisher
Thousand Oaks ▪ London ▪ New Delhi

For information:

Sage Publications, Inc.
2455 Teller Road
Thousand Oaks, California 91320
E-mail: order@sagepub.com

Sage Publications Ltd.
6 Bonhill Street
London EC2A 4PU
United Kingdom

Sage Publications India Pvt. Ltd.
M-32 Market
Greater Kailash I
New Delhi 110 048 India

Printed in the United States of America

Library of Congress Cataloging-in-Publication Data

Redman, Barbara Klug.
   Measurement Instruments in Clinical Ethics / by Barbara Redman.
      p. cm.
   Includes bibliographical references and index.
   ISBN 0-7619-1517-6 (c: acid paper)—ISBN 0-7619-1518-4 (p: acid paper)
   1. Medical ethics—Research—Methodology. 2. Psychometrics. I. Title.
   R725.5 .R43 2001
   174'.2—dc21   2001001019

02   03   04   05   06   07   08   7   6   5   4   3   2   1

Acquiring Editor:	C. Deborah Laughton
Editorial Assistant:	Veronica Novak
Production Editor:	Claudia A. Hoffman
Editorial Assistant:	Cindy Bear
Typesetters:	Denyse Dunn/Tina Hill
Indexer:	Molly Hall
Cover Designer:	Michelle Lee

Contents

Preface

The evolution of ethical issues in clinical and research work in health care has accelerated significantly. Such concerns include the struggle toward patient autonomy in end-of-life decisions and subjects' access to rational but subjective choices for particular arms of a clinical trial. Practitioners are searching for coherent and defensible answers to guide their conduct in a dramatically changing environment.

Although ethical debates are grounded in philosophy, empirical studies of key assumptions and consequences are now reported in the health literature. An important aspect of clarifying these assumptions and consequences is the development of measurement instruments in which psychometric characteristics have been well studied. Many studies of ethical concepts in clinical and research activities use interview scales or other methods of gathering data that have not undergone rigorous analysis of their psychometric characteristics. But some have.

This book presents a number of these instruments and describes and critiques their stages of development. Its purpose is to play a small role in furthering the debate about what evolving ethical standards mean for clinicians and researchers. It does not include instruments to measure moral development in individuals (including health professionals) or describe the methods of economic appraisal and valuation of health states because these have been adequately dealt with elsewhere (Ketefian, 1989; Newbold, 1995; Rest & Narvaez, 1994).

REFERENCES

Ketefian, S. (1989). Moral reasoning and ethical practice in nursing: Measurement issues. *Nursing Clinics of North America, 24*, 509-521.

Newbold, D. (1995). A brief description of the methods of economic appraisal and the valuation of health states. *Journal of Advanced Nursing, 21*, 325-333.

Rest, J. R., & Narvaez, D. (Eds). (1994). *Moral development in the professions: Psychology and applied ethics.* Hillsdale, NJ: Lawrence Erlbaum.

1

Empirical Studies in Ethics and Psychometric Standards for Measurement

Ethics is a branch of philosophy that attempts to critically examine human conduct, focusing on right and wrong, the good or the harm of actions. Bioethics focuses on applied ethical inquiry into all situations in which biology affects human affairs; medical ethics is a narrower term referring to applied ethics in the medical realm (Grodin, 1995). With its major scholarly traditions in theology and philosophy, much of the published work in bioethics has consisted of theoretical discussions of ethical concepts or analyses of case discussions. During the late 1980s, empirical studies of the context and management of ethical issues in health settings began to appear (Arnold & Forrow, 1993). These studies clarify how ethical standards are being defined and implemented in care or research settings, and identify which ethical theories or standards need to be further developed.

There is a ferment in applying ethical standards to practice, which is only partly related to dramatic changes in health care organization and financing throughout the world. Although new rules about the flow of money have raised significant issues about provider conflicts of interest and the fairness of new patterns of allocation of health care resources, other movements such as care reform in the quality of dying seem only marginally related to financial reform. Application of new ethical standards to care and research requires precise measurement instruments that have not previously existed in this field.

1

Instruments embody particular definitions of an issue and particular standards in the interpretation of their scores that then focus the debate about a specific ethical issue. The use of measurement instruments allows everyone to determine how their practice conforms to evolving standards and to participate in the debate about what those standards should be. Use of the instruments engages people in fields with scientific traditions of measurement in ways they might otherwise never consider ethical issues. Distinct definitions and instrumentation are essential to a universal change of standards of ethical practice.

DEVELOPMENT OF MEASUREMENT INSTRUMENTS IN CLINICAL AND RESEARCH ETHICS

The development of measurement instruments in clinical and research ethics is just beginning. Although they are difficult to retrieve from the literature and thus to assure that one has been inclusive, many of the instruments retrieved for this book focus on issues of patient autonomy and preference. This emphasis reflects the ongoing project of moving from provider-generated decisions to those in which patients are participants or at least to decisions that are consistent with patient values. This evolving set of measurement instruments should help us traverse the next phase of this task by giving practitioners an understanding of the distribution of preferences. This is also a field in which the direction of the evolving standard is clear (more patient autonomy), although the appropriate point on the autonomy continuum remains debated. This kind of measure is also consistent with psychometric traditions because it measures a psychological characteristic of individuals.

In other areas of bioethics such as justice, few measurement instruments are available and yet are already greatly needed. Disruptions in the flow of health care resources have generated many concerns about fairness between individuals in health plans and between groups different on such morally relevant characteristics as gender and race. Many such questions will be raised as the levels of equity (fair and equal access to quality health care) achieved in many countries from the 1950s through the 1980s are endangered or have disappeared (Callahan, 1998). Whereas measurement approaches to the allocation of resources have been developed in economics, in philosophical orientation they are largely consequential, and their methods are difficult for the ordinary practitioner to understand and to use. However, analyses of the results from common measurement instruments such as those for health status to address issues of distributive justice are available (Clayton & Williams, 1994).

This book focuses on instruments that measure explicitly ethical concepts or other closely related concepts, and that are useful in clinical settings or in research on clinical issues. It does not include instruments that measure moral development, including moral reasoning of health professionals; this is a separate literature. It also does not include measurement of attitudes of health professionals or the public toward ethical issues. On average, attitudes account for a small percentage of the variance in behavior, and summaries of relevant research conclude that attitudes should not be used as an easily measured substitute for behavior (Kraus, 1995).

In addition to a broad reading of the ethics and clinical literature, instruments were retrieved from Bioethicsline by searches under the terms "informed consent," "patient preference," "competence," "health care rationing," "patient selection," "ethics," "study," or "empirical research," covering sources published between 1989 and 1998. Unpublished materials such as dissertations were not included. All citations obtained from Bioethicsline were screened for measurement instruments for which at least some psychometric information was available and through citation indexes for other studies that had used the instruments. If the instruments were not included in published sources, copies and available psychometric information were requested from authors. Some authors refused to provide instruments or had already licensed them, or did not respond to multiple contacts and so their instruments could not be included. Thus, the 30 instruments included in this book are most certainly an incomplete list.

Instruments were very difficult to retrieve and to date there seems to be no focused attention on issues for the measurement of ethical concepts. In some areas such as competence, the most completely developed instrument has already been made available in detailed publication elsewhere (Grisso & Applebaum, 1998). Measurement problems abound. Most instruments are in very early stages of development with minimal information available about their measurement characteristics. This means that at the very least, users must collect information about instrument validity and reliability as part of their studies. Additional problems are related to the methods used to study ethical constructs and to the pace of development of the field. For example, vignettes are commonly used to portray contextual detail surrounding ethical issues. Most authors of instruments containing vignettes provide some evidence that the hypothetical situations and associated response options represent those faced by patients. What is less frequently provided is evidence that the measurements that result generalize to actual patient behaviors in real situations.

A second problem is that measurement instruments address only a portion of the elements of an important ethical construct. For example, Sugarman, McCrory, and Hubal's (1998) review of 99 studies of informed consent showed a substantial amount of literature related to understanding informed consent, in contrast to other aspects of this construct such as voluntariness. Although this presumably occurs because the former is easier to measure, it leaves the user in the position of being unable to measure precisely and ultimately to assure that all elements of informed consent are met.

STANDARDS FOR INSTRUMENT DEVELOPMENT

The process of instrument development and validation seeks information about the plausibility of the results of measurement. Does the instrument consistently yield more or less the same results when administered on several occasions to stable participants, across raters, or with the same rater at different times, or with parallel forms of the test (reliability)? Is the instrument actually measuring what it is supposed to measure—all relevant aspects of the domain or area (content validity)? Do scores from the instrument relate to other measures in the way one would expect if they are measuring what they are supposed to measure or support hypotheses based on theory (construct validity)? Does an instrument designed to measure change in people over time, including responses to an intervention, detect minimal meaningful differences (responsiveness, also called sensitivity)(Guyatt, Walter, & Norman, 1987)? Well-established sources (McDowell & Newell, 1996) describe conceptual and technical aspects of measurement including the psychometric methods on which instruments in this book are based, and suggest standards for reliability and validity. These include

Reliability. Internal consistency is a measure of homogeneity of items in a scale. For continuous measures, Cronbach's alpha values between .70 and .90 are acceptable (in the middle .90s for use with individuals). Correlation of an item with the total score of the scale to which it belongs (item-total correlations) should exceed .20.

Test-retest reliability should be in the .70 to .80 range (Lamping, Rowe, Clarke, Black, & Lessof, 1998).

Validity. Describes the range of interpretations that can appropriately be placed on a measurement score. More formally, validity is an integrated evaluative judgment of the degree to which empirical evidence and theoretical rationales support the adequacy and appropriateness of inferences and actions based on test scores or other modes of assessment. Validation is a continuing process (Messick, 1989).

Content validity is evaluated logically by consensus of patient and expert opinion, reviews of literature and of existing instruments.

Criterion validity is the correlation between the measure and a gold standard measure of the same attribute, both given at the same time. Validity for predictions for groups of people should be between .60 and .70 and predictions for individuals should be .80.

Construct validity assesses the extent to which the instrument measures the attribute it purports to measure. Aspects are convergent and discriminate validity; is the instrument able to detect differences in groups known to be similar or different in the attribute being measured?

Factor analysis reduces a set of variables (instrument items) to smaller clusters of correlated items called factors. The content of the items within a factor and the mathematical weights of factors are used to define the concept or support prior theorizing about its nature. Factor analysis is used to define subscales and to refine the instrument by eliminating items (McDowell & Newell, 1996).

Responsiveness. Ability to detect subtle but significant clinical change. This characteristic is determined by serial administration of the measure at different points over time when clinical changes are expected to occur, and in comparison with other criteria of change. Rasch analysis is a specialized analysis not yet commonly used in health scales that shows where each patient fits along the measurement scale. It indicates how consistently the relationships among the items hold in different subgroups of respondents (McDowell & Newell, 1996).

Clinimetrics provides a reminder that subjective data from phenomena in clinical care such as human sensations and reactions are important and worth pursuing. An approach to developing rigorous measurement instruments based on clinimetrics may be found in Feinstein (1987).

There has long been a concern about the social consequences of the use of measurement instruments, sometimes classified as consequential validity. In other words, despite other supportive evidence, the validity of an instrument can be in question if its use, including score interpretation, yields harmful consequences such as reinforcing social inequities, altering conceptions of individual identity, or enhancing societal or institutional ability to monitor and control people's actions. Because these harmful consequences can be intended or unintended, it is necessary to monitor the repercussions of the use of test results (Messick, 1989).

An early way to identify potential problems is to analyze value implications in the construct label, in the theory underlying test interpretation, and the ideologies in which the theory is embedded. In addition, using the results of a measurement instrument necessitates setting a performance standard of some kind, which may be unrealistic for some individuals especially if, as is commonly the case, instrument development has been accomplished with only a narrow segment of the population with which it will be used. The following set of questions could be used as screening questions for consequential validity:

1. What standard is inherent in the measure—is it fair or will it deny autonomy to some groups of people?

2. Has the potential for cultural, medical, and gender bias been disproved?

3. Are there procedural safeguards and other sources of information to be used in making the judgments so that information from a faulty tool can be identified and not be used in a damaging way?

4. Is use of the instrument better than the current way decisions are made—more accurate and clearer? Are the potential social consequences worse or better than not testing at all?

5. Are there efficacious interventions to deal with problems described by the measurement instrument? Are they available to the clients? If not, will use of the instrument set up expectations that cannot be met or create a problem for which there is no solution or help to reach a solution?

In general, what are the intended and unintended social consequences of test use? If the consequences are adverse for some groups, it is essential to know if these consequences are linked to sources of test invalidity such as being based on a construct or theory that is culturally biased. Viewing any situation through multiple value positions is helpful. Further detail on validity, including consequential validity, may be found in Messick (1989).

SUMMARY

The use of instruments to measure ethical constructs seems to be accelerating but is still in the early stages of development. For many instruments, information about the basic measurement characteristics described above is still being collected. In addition, development is uneven across the field and within ethical constructs. Yet, careful development and use of measurement instruments in this field can be very helpful in applying evolving ethical standards in practice and research.

DESCRIPTION OF INSTRUMENTS

Instruments are clustered by topics. The first set of topics relates to patient preference, patient comprehension, and decisional capacity. The second topic is advance directives, with instruments relating both to patients and to providers. The third topic relates to providers' choices: withdrawal of life support, ethical environment for practice, moral sensitivity, aggressiveness of care, and recipient selection. The final cluster reflects general issues for health professionals.

Each instrument is reviewed within a common framework of description, psychometric properties, and summary and critique. Permission to reprint all of the instruments was granted, which in most instances was provided by the authors who developed them.

DEFINITIONS

Autonomy is a moral obligation to respect self-determination.

Beneficence is a moral obligation to do good for others.

Bioethics focuses on applied ethical inquiry into all situations in which biology affects human affairs.

Ethics is a branch of philosophy that focuses on the rightness or wrongness of actions.

Instrument is a measuring device for determining the present value of a quantity under observation.

Justice is a moral obligation to treat others fairly.

Non-maleficence is a moral obligation not to inflict evil or harm.

Vignette is a short descriptive sketch describing an incident or situation.

REFERENCES

Arnold, R. M., & Forrow, L. (1993). Empirical research in medical ethics: An introduction. *Theoretical Medicine, 14,* 195-196.

Bioethicsline. Available: bioethicsline.georgetown.edu/bioline.htm.

Callahan, D. (1998). *False hopes.* New York: Simon & Schuster.

Clayton, M. G., & Williams, A. D. (1994). Subjective health assessment and distributive justice. In C. Jenkinson (Ed.), *Measuring health and medical outcomes.* London: University College London.

Feinstein, A. R. (1987). *Clinimetrics.* New Haven, CT: Yale University Press.

Grisso, T., & Applebaum, P. S. (1998). *Assessing competence to consent to treatment.* New York: Oxford University Press.

Grodin, M. A. (Ed.). (1995). *Meta medical ethics.* Boston: Kluwer Academic.

Guyatt, G., Walter, S., & Norman, G. (1987). Measuring change over time: Assessing the usefulness of evaluative instruments. *Journal of Chronic Disease, 40,* 171-178.

Kraus, S. J. (1995). Attitudes and the prediction of behavior: A meta-analysis of the empirical literature. *Personality and Social Psychology Bulletin, 21,* 58-75.

Lamping, D. L., Rowe, P., Clarke, A., Black, N., & Lessof, L. (1998). Development and validation of the menorrhagia outcomes questionnaire. *British Journal of Obstetrics & Gynaecology, 105,* 766-779.

McDowell, I., & Newell, C. (1996). *Measuring health* (2nd ed.). New York: Oxford University Press.

Messick, S. (1989). Validity. In R. L. Linn (Ed.), *Educational measurement* (3rd ed.). New York: Macmillan.

Sugarman, J., McCrory, D. C., & Hubal, R. C. (1998). Getting meaningful informed consent from older adults: A structural review of empirical research. *Journal of the American Geriatrics Society, 46,* 517-524.

2 Patient Preference

The preferences of patients, based on their own values and personal assessments of benefits and burdens, are ethically and legally relevant in all health care. These preferences reflect the value of personal autonomy and are expressed clinically in accommodation (where possible) to that patient's needs and preferences and more formally in informed consent. When faced with the same clinical situations, different patients may express quite distinct but reasonable preferences, desired levels of autonomy, and involvement in care as may another patient at different times in his or her illness. Likewise, providers vary widely in their views about the appropriate role of patients in decision making about care and about particular choices such as life support, which in many instances reflects the beliefs of their different professions. Providers inferring patient preferences without formal assessment frequently get them wrong (Charles, Gafni, & Whelan, 1997).

The instruments that follow provide a structured way to assess patient preferences for preferred overall level of involvement in decision making about their care and for particular momentous decisions (cardiopulmonary resuscitation, life support, life-sustaining treatments). These preferences are then used within the provider-patient relationship to construct choices and a plan of care as well as a basis for policy development. They provide an opportunity to describe and understand differences in what providers assume patients prefer and patients' actual preferences and to study the degree to which patient preferences are actually carried out in clinical situations. Arguments for or against patient autonomy have generally been based on normative ethical reasoning alone.

The goal of interventions to increase patients' participation in health care is to reach an ideal model of shared patient-provider decision making. These instruments may be helpful in documenting some of the outcomes from such interventions.

REFERENCE

Charles, C., Gafni, A., & Whelan, T. (1997). Shared decision-making in the medical encounter: What does it mean? *Social Science & Medicine, 44,* 681-692.

THE AUTONOMY PREFERENCE INDEX (API)

Developed by Jack Ende, Lewis Kazis,
Arlene Ash, and Mark A. Moskowitz

INSTRUMENT DEVELOPMENT, ADMINISTRATION, AND SCORING

Although patients typically express high preferences for information about their illness and its treatment, their preferences for participation in treatment decision making are much more diversely distributed. The Autonomy Preference Index (API) consists of an 8-item scale on information seeking and a 15-item scale on decision making. The latter scale has six general items and nine items related to three clinical vignettes representing different levels of illness severity: upper respiratory tract illness representing mild disease, hypertension representing moderate disease, and myocardial infarction representing severe or most threatening disease (Ende, Kazis, Ash, & Moskowitz, 1989). Strongest preferences in favor of decision or information seeking are assigned scores of 5, and weakest preferences show scores of 1; scores for each scale are summed over items.

PSYCHOMETRIC PROPERTIES

The API was constructed based on a Delphi study of clinicians, medical sociologists, and ethicists. Patients' preferences for making decisions and their desire for information emerged as the two most important dimensions for differentiating patients who seek an active role in their care from those who prefer a more passive role. Items were field-tested and reviewed with patients to ensure content validity.

The API was tested with 312 patients randomly selected from a hospital-based primary care clinic in a university medical center. The decision-making scale correlated significantly and positively with global questions about the amount of control patients wanted, providing support for concurrent validity. People with diabetes selected by staff as being highly motivated and adept at self-care scored significantly higher on the decision-making scale than did the general study population, supporting convergent validity. Factor analysis supported the two scales as different dimensions of patients' attitudes toward autonomy (Ende et al., 1989). Test-retest reliability was .84 for the decision-making scale and .83 for the information-seeking scale. Each scale had a Cronbach's alpha of .82, a measure of internal consistency.

Among patients at the primary care clinic, the mean score for information seeking on a 0- to 100-point scale was 79.5 with a variance of 11.5. On the decision-making scale, where 0 signified no desired involvement and 100 complete patient control, the mean score for the study population was 33.2 ± 12.5. Patients preferred more decision-making power during minor illness than during major illness. Patients' preferences should therefore be regarded as dynamic as their conditions and situations change (Ende et al., 1989).

Items from the API have been used in several studies. They generally support and elaborate on the findings of Ende et al. (1989). Ghali, Freund, Boss, Ryan, & Moskowitz (1997) found scores among women and their physicians considering hormone replacement therapy at menopause to be similar on the several API items used as did Ende et al. (1989). Thompson, Pitts, and Schwankovsky (1993) used only the API vignettes section. Catalon et al. (1994) also used a modified API to study differences between male patients with HIV infection and their providers. Common HIV-related problems replaced the conditions included in the original instrument. Ende et al. found that staff had higher preference for patient involvement in decision making than did the patients themselves. The opposite was the case for information seeking. The API scores were highest for social workers, followed by nurses and patients, with physicians lowest of all and significantly different from both nurses and social workers. Among patients, disease progression was associated with a reduction in patients' wishes for decision making. Evidence regarding reliability and validity was not collected as part of this study. Deber, Kraet-schmer, and Irvine (1996) also found scores of 81.39 (on a 100-point scale) on the information subscale of the API, which had a Cronbach's alpha of only .11. Because each of these studies modified the instrument, they provide no further information about the validity of the API for various uses.

SUMMARY AND CRITIQUE

Using the API, Ende et al. (1989) found that patients' preferences for decision making were weak, especially in serious illness. In contrast, they had strong interest in being well informed. A number of studies have found that the mean level of desired involvement in decision making is strongly on the side of more physician control rather than patient control. Thompson et al. (1993) showed that this may not be the case with decisions that patients feel qualified to evaluate and suggest that most of the items on the API refer to decisions that require medical expertise. These authors found that respondents expressed more desire for involvement in decisions not requiring medical knowledge, and thus challenge the conclusions of other studies that patients in general do not want to participate. Because patients make informed choices that involve a more comprehensive variety of factors than physicians typically consider, decisions in which they are involved are more likely to be appropriate. Others (Deber et al., 1996) used portions of the API in a study of 300 patients undergoing angiography. They suggest that the API is not clearly defined. They also charge that it contains a mixture of problem-solving and decision-making elements, which also inclines patients to defer to physicians because they do not have the expert knowledge to solve the problems.

Procedures for development of the complete content domain of patient autonomy, description of that complete domain, and the basis on which the two elements of patient autonomy included in the API were chosen are superficially described (Ende et al., 1989). Given the continued controversy in the field about the definition of patient autonomy, such clarification would be helpful. Although still minimal, the API does present more complete evidence supporting validity than does almost any other instrument described in this book. Identified uses of the API have been for research. Because it is likely that users would frequently alter the content of the vignettes, comparison across studies producing information about validity of the scales will be difficult. In addition, although the title includes the term "autonomy," there are many senses in which the autonomy of preferences is used that are not included.

The API, of course, does not provide information about the rightfulness of patient autonomy as a guiding ethical principle. Neither does it provide a way to obtain patient preferences for particular situations. Yet, instruments approaching the measurement of autonomy and preference are important because in their absence, the direction for appropriate level of autonomy is based on general normative ethical reasoning alone. Such reasoning may not reflect actual patient preferences and may delay the reform of practices to the level of autonomy that patients desire.

REFERENCES

Catalon, J., Brener, H., Andrews, H., Day, A., Cullum, S., Hooker, M.. & Gazzard, B. (1994). Whose health is it? Views about decision-making and information-seeking from people with HIV infection and their professional careers. *AIDS Care, 6*, 349-356.

Deber, R. B., Kraetschmer, N., & Irvine, J. (1996). What role do patients wish to play in treatment decision making? *Archives of Internal Medicine, 156*, 1414-1420.

Ende, J., Kazis, L., Ash, A., & Moskowitz, M. A. (1989). Measuring patients' desire for autonomy. *Journal of General Internal Medicine, 4*, 23-30.

Ghali, W. A., Freund, K. M., Boss, R. D., Ryan, C. A., & Moskowitz, M. A. (1997). Menopausal hormone therapy: Physician awareness of patient attitudes. *American Journal of Medicine, 103*, 3-10.

Thompson, S. C., Pitts, J. S., & Schwankovsky, L. (1993). Preferences for involvement in medical decision-making: Situational and demographic influences. *Patient Education and Counseling, 22*, 133-140.

Instrument 2.1

THE AUTONOMY PREFERENCE INDEX (API)*

I. Decision making preference scale
   A. General items for decision making preference. (Patients respond to each item on a five-point Likert scale. Response choices range from "strongly disagree" to "strongly agree.")

       1.† The important medical decisions should be made by your doctor, not by you.

       2. You should go along with your doctor's advice even if you disagree with it.

       3.† When hospitalized, you should *NOT* be making decisions about your own care

       4. You should feel free to make decisions about everyday medical problems.

       5.† If you were sick, as your illness became worse you would want your doctor to take greater control.

       6. You should decide how frequently you need a check-up.

   B. Vignettes. (Patients respond to each item on a five-point scale. Response choices are: "you alone," "mostly you," "the doctor and you equally," "mostly the doctor," and "the doctor alone."

Upper Respiratory Tract Illness. "Suppose you developed a sore throat, stuffy nose, and cough that lasted for three days. You are about to call your doctor on the telephone. Who should make the following decisions?"

---

    7. Whether you should be seen by the doctor.

    8. Whether a chest x-ray should be taken.

    9. Whether you should try taking cough syrup.

High Blood Pressure. "Suppose you went to your doctor for a routine physical examination and he or she found that everything was all right except that your blood pressure was high (170/100). Who should make the following decisions?"

---

    10. When the next visit to check your blood pressure should be.

    11. Whether you should take some time off from work to relax.

    12. Whether you should be treated with medication or diet.

> **Myocardial Infarction.** "Suppose you had an attack of severe chest pain that lasted for almost an hour, frightening you enough so that you went to the emergency room. In the emergency room the doctors discover that you are having a heart attack. Your own doctor is called and you are taken up to the intensive care unit. Who should make the following decisions?"

    13. How often the nurses should wake you up to check your temperature and blood pressure.

    14. Whether you may have visitors aside from your immediate family.

    15. Whether a cardiologist should be consulted.

II. Information-seeking preference scale
    A. Items for information-seeking preference. (Patients respond on a five-point Likert scale. Response choices range from "strongly disagree" to "strongly agree.")
        16. As you become sicker you should be told more and more about your illness.
        17. You should understand completely what is happening inside your body as a result of your illness.
        18. Even if the news is bad, you should be well informed.
        19. Your doctor should explain the purpose of your laboratory tests.
        20. You should be given information only when you ask for it.
        21. It is important for you to know all the side effects of your medication.
        22. Information about your illness is as important to you as treatment.
        23. When there is more than one method to treat a problem, you should be told about each one.

SOURCE: From "Measuring patients' desire for autonomy," by J. Ende, L. Kazis, A. Ash, and M. A. Moskowitz, 1989, *Journal of General Internal Medicine, 4,* pp. 23-30. Reprinted by permission of Blackwell Science, Inc.
*A copy of the API in the format used for administration to subjects is available from the authors.
†Scoring for these items is reversed, and goes from 5 to 1, rather than 1 to 5.

INFORMATION STYLES QUESTIONNAIRE (ISQ)

Developed by Barrie Cassileth, Robert V. Zupkis,
Katherine Sutton-Smith, and Vicki March

INSTRUMENT DEVELOPMENT, ADMINISTRATION, AND SCORING

The ISQ examines cancer patients' attitudes about information and participation in medical decisions. Literature on informed consent is primarily focused on patients who seek detailed information and prefer to participate in their own care. Patients who want a minimum of information and who do not want to participate in treatment decisions also should be served by this doctrine. The ISQ offers a way to determine participation preferences and what patients perceive as necessary information and as undesired information (Cassileth, Zupkis, Sutton-Smith, & March, 1980).

The ISQ has been used in research to study information preferences of patients undergoing autologous bone marrow transplantation (ABMT)—a procedure that imposes increased demands for disclosure of information to assure informed consent. In this pilot study with 27 Caucasian, well-educated patients, 90% preferred maximum amounts of detailed information (Fisch et al., 1998).

The 12 items associated with question 3 are scored with 1 = absolutely need, 2 = like to have, and 3 = do not want, with the information style score being the sum of these items. The lowest possible score (12) for this item indicates the strongest desire for information and the highest possible score (36) indicates an aversion to information.

PSYCHOMETRIC PROPERTIES

The ISQ evolved from a series of pilot tests with 50 patients; it uses wording that patients found comprehensible and was found to discriminate between patients' viewpoints. The ISQ was tested with 256 outpatients attending hematology/oncology and radiation therapy clinics and with inpatients with metatastic disease in one teaching hospital (Cassileth et al., 1980). Response patterns for the amount of information patients wanted on specific items may be found in Cassileth et al.

SUMMARY AND CRITIQUE

Cassileth et al. note that the very topic of the ISQ may be harmful for patients who cope with illness by denial or by avoiding information. A strong correlation between preferences for maximum information and desire to participate in decisions suggested that information style and participation preference represent components of a single attitudinal approach. The original study also showed strong positive relationships between patients' preferences for active involvement in their own care and wanting as much knowledge as possible and hopefulness. This finding does not support the old notion that physicians' sharing knowledge would have the side effect of destroying hope.

The study by Fisch et al. (1998) provides evidence to debunk another myth—that the provision of complex information needed to make treatment decisions would foster patient psychological distress. In both the Cassileth et al. (1980) and the Fisch et al. (1998) studies, participants demonstrated with the ISQ a clear avidity for information.

Comprehensive information on validity and reliability could not be located, and scoring protocols are incomplete. Yet, the research using the ISQ has addressed questions important to the ideology of informed consent. It would seem useful to replicate available studies using diverse populations but at the same time performing basic validity and reliability work.

REFERENCES

Cassileth, B. R., Zupkis, R. V., Sutton-Smith, K., & March, V. (1980). Information and participation preferences among cancer patients. *Annals of Internal Medicine, 92,* 832-836.

Fisch, M., Unverzagt, F., Hanna, M., Bledsoe, P., Menke, C., & Cornetta, K. (1998). Information preferences, reading ability, and emotional changes in outpatients during the process of obtaining informed consent for autologous bone-marrow transplantation. *Journal of Cancer Education, 13,* 71-75.

Instrument 2.2

PATIENT INFORMATION QUESTIONNAIRE

Date_____

Age: ____ years   Race: ( ) White   ( ) Oriental   ( ) Black   ( ) Hispanic
Sex: ( ) M   ( ) F   ( ) Other _____

Education: (Circle or check highest grade completed):
    Elementary grades   1   2   3   4   5   6   7   8
    High School   9   10   11   12
    ( ) Vocational training
    ( ) Some college
    ( ) College graduate
    ( ) Post-graduate studies

What is your diagnosis? _____

How long have you known about your present illness? _____

Which of the following kinds of treatment have you received for your present
illness (circle all that apply):

    A. Surgery   C. Radiation Therapy
    B. Chemotherapy   D. Other (please explain)

---

1. *After they have all the information they need* about their illness and treatment, some patients prefer not to get any more details, and others prefer
   to get additional information. Please circle the statement that best describes your preference:

A	B	C	D	E
No more details	A few	Some more	Many more	As many more
than needed	more details	details	details	details as possible

2. Which statement best described *your* point of view? (circle one)

   A. I prefer to leave decisions about my medical care and treatment
      up to my doctor.

   B. I prefer to participate in decisions about my medical care and
      treatment.

3. Here are some types of information about your illness. For each one, please indicate whether you absolutely need this information, would like to have it, or do not want it:

	I absolutely need this information	I would like to have this information	I do not want this information
A. What the specific name of the medical illness is	( )	( )	( )
B. What the treatment will accomplish	( )	( )	( )
C. What the day-to-day (or week-to-week) progress is	( )	( )	( )
D. Whether or not it is cancer	( )	( )	( )
E. Exactly what the treatment will do inside my body	( )	( )	( )
F. What all the possible side effects are	( )	( )	( )
G. How effective the treatment has been for other patients	( )	( )	( )
H. Whether all parts of the body are involved	( )	( )	( )
I. Whether it is inherited or contagious	( )	( )	( )
J. What the likelihood of cure is	( )	( )	( )
K. Examples of cases where the treatment has been effective	( )	( )	( )
L. Examples of cases where the treatment has not been effective	( )	( )	( )

4. Is there any other information you feel you need?

   ( ) No   Yes (please explain): _____

   _____

5. Which of the following diseases reminds you most of cancer? (please circle one)
   A. Heart disease
   B. Kidney disease
   C. Mental illness
   D. Leprosy
   E. Multiple sclerosis

6. If you were talking about this illness, which phrase would you most often use?
   A. The Big C
   B. Cancer
   C. Tumor
   D. It
   E. Other:_____

7. Do your friends know what your exact diagnosis is?
   (please circle one letter)

   A. No
   B. Yes, but only my most intimate friends
   C. Yes, most of my friends and neighbors

   Comments: _____

8. Which statement best reflects your attitude toward information about
   your illness?

   A. I want *only* information needed to care for myself properly
   B. I want additional information only if it is good news
   C. I want as much information as possible, good and bad

   Please explain your choice: _____
   _____

Thank you very much for your help!

SOURCE: © Barrie R. Cassileth, Ph.D., 20 Holsberry Road, Box 222, Truro, MA 02666 USA;
BarrieC@juno.com. Reprinted with permission.

DECISION INVOLVEMENT QUESTIONNAIRE (DIQ)

*Developed by Suzanne C. Thompson,
Jennifer S. Pitts, and Lenore Schwankovsky*

INSTRUMENT DEVELOPMENT, ADMINISTRATION, AND SCORING

On the one hand, dissatisfaction with the traditional approach to doctor-patient interaction has led professionals and patients alike to search for partnership models in which patients work with physicians to determine the form of medical treatment. On the other hand, a number of studies have found that the mean level of desired involvement in decision making rests strongly on the side of more physician rather than more patient control. Several instruments reviewed in this book have been developed to understand this point of balance in various situations.

Items in the Autonomy Preference Index (API; reviewed elsewhere in this book) refer to decisions that require medical expertise, such as whether a cardiologist should be consulted following a myocardial infarction. The Decision Involvement Questionnaire (DIQ) was developed to tap desire for input in situations in which medical expertise is not required. The four vignettes describe medical problems of varying severity, each requiring treatment but in which there are two treatment choices. Each choice is equally appropriate medically but differs in effects on the patient's lifestyle, side effects likely to be experienced, or the trade-off between quality and length of life. Scores of the items are summed (Thompson, Pitts, & Schwankovsky, 1993).

PSYCHOMETRIC PROPERTIES

The DIQ was tested with 459 members of an HMO who were largely white and female with some college education, and a median income of $30,000. Internal reliability (Cronbach's alpha) was .87. The DIQ showed expected patterns of relationship with other measures of involvement. It correlated more strongly with the Autonomy Preference Index than with the Behavioral Involvement subscale of the Health Opinion Scale, a measure of preference for self-care rather than physician treatment. These findings support construct validity with evidence of convergent and discriminant validity. As also might be predicted, respondents expressed more desire for involvement in decisions not requiring medical knowledge (DIQ) than they did for decisions requiring such information (API), supporting the need for a separate scale (Thompson et al., 1993).

SUMMARY AND CRITIQUE

The DIQ was developed to test patient desire for involvement in decisions that do not require medical expertise. It has thus far been used in research to determine the situations in which patients feel competent to be more autonomous in decision making. Because such participation has been associated with better patient outcomes (e.g., less discomfort, greater alleviation of symptoms; Thompson et al., 1993), it seems to benefit patients beyond its value in matching patient attitudes and values to treatment options.

Formal analysis of content validity appears not to have been done. Although the population studied was homogeneous, beginning evidence of validity and reliability is available.

REFERENCE

Thompson, S. C., Pitts, J. S., & Schwankovsky, L. (1993). Preferences for involvement in medical decision-making: Situational and demographic influences. *Patient Education & Counseling, 22,* 133-140.

Instrument 2.3

DECISION INVOLVEMENT QUESTIONNAIRE

For the following scenarios, try to imagine yourself in each situation. Then indicate who you think should decide which treatment program you should receive: you alone, mostly you, the doctor and you equally, mostly the doctor, or the doctor alone.

Suppose you fall and seriously injure your knee. There are two treatment programs that are medically appropriate for your condition. You can either have surgery that will be painful and require bed rest for a month OR you can enter a twice-a-week rehabilitation program for a year. Both have a 90% chance of success.

Who should decide which treatment program you receive?

The doctor alone	Mostly the doctor	The doctor and you equally	Mostly you	You alone
1	2	3	4	5

Suppose your doctor tells you that you have high blood pressure. Two treatment choices are possible. One is medication that has possible effects of dizziness, weight gain, and impotence. The second is to adhere to a low-salt diet that involves restricting many of your favorite foods. Both have been found to be moderately successful.

Who should decide which treatment program you receive?

The doctor alone	Mostly the doctor	The doctor and you equally	Mostly you	You alone
1	2	3	4	5

Suppose your doctor discovers that you have a cancerous growth. There are two surgical treatments available. One is to have extensive surgery which would be disfiguring, but would most likely remove all the cancer. The second is to have minor surgery that would not be disfiguring, but would require follow-up chemotherapy that may have side effects of nausea, hair loss, and fatigue.

Who should decide which treatment program you receive?

The doctor alone	Mostly the doctor	The doctor and you equally	Mostly you	You alone
1	2	3	4	5

Suppose you visit your doctor because you start having occasional stress headaches. There are two ways to treat your headaches. One is for the doctor to give you a powerful medication that will eliminate the pain but make you too drowsy to be able to work. The other is to attend four stress reduction classes.

Who should decide which treatment program you receive?

The doctor alone	Mostly the doctor	The doctor and you equally	Mostly you	You alone
1	2	3	4	5

Suppose that you have a chronic illness that is painful. It could be treated with strong pain medication that would leave you groggy and might worsen your condition in the long run OR you could not treat the pain and just live with it.

Who should decide which treatment program you receive?

The doctor alone	Mostly the doctor	The doctor and you equally	Mostly you	You alone
1	2	3	4	5

Suppose that you were diagnosed with a kidney condition. A new drug treatment was available that is very effective but has been known to cause heart irregularities and permanent vision problems in some patients. The other alternative is to have standard treatment—it won't cure you but will manage the problem with few side effects.

Who should decide which treatment program you receive?

The doctor alone	Mostly the doctor	The doctor and you equally	Mostly you	You alone
1	2	3	4	5

Suppose you developed an upper respiratory infection. A new antibiotic is available—it works in a short time, but requires you to wake up several times during the night to take medication. The other choice is to have the standard treatment—it will take longer to knock out the infection, but you do not need to disturb your sleep.

Who should decide which treatment program you receive?

The doctor alone	Mostly the doctor	The doctor and you equally	Mostly you	You alone
1	2	3	4	5

Suppose you have surgery and need to take pain medication for a week to control pain from your incision. Two choices for pain administration are available: a pain control machine by the side of your bed that allows you to push a button to get a dose of pain medication at regular intervals OR the usual situation where you call the nurse when you need more medication. Who should decide which method of getting pain medication should be used?

Who should decide which treatment program you receive?

The doctor alone	Mostly the doctor	The doctor and you equally	Mostly you	You alone
1	2	3	4	5

Suppose you have a history of heart problems and have been having recurring episodes of moderately severe heart pain. There are two methods available for treating your condition: an invasive procedure involving some risk and discomfort OR a long-term modified and restrictive diet.

Who should decide which treatment program you receive?

The doctor alone	Mostly the doctor	The doctor and you equally	Mostly you	You alone
1	2	3	4	5

SOURCE: S. C. Thompson, J. S. Pitts, and L. Schwankovsky. Reprinted with permission from pom-vms1.pomona.edu/~sthompson/diq1.htm

DESIRE FOR LENGTH OF BENEFIT SCALE (DLBS) DESIRE FOR PROBABLE BENEFIT SCALE (DPBS)

Developed by Marion Danis, Elizabeth Mutran, Joanne M. Garrett, Sally C. Stearns, Rebecca T. Slifkin, Laura Hanson, Jude F. Williams, and Larry R. Churchill

INSTRUMENT DEVELOPMENT, ADMINISTRATION, AND SCORING

It is now understood that life-sustaining treatment decisions should be made in keeping with patient preferences. At the same time, we have a very incomplete understanding of the views of the critically ill on prolonging life or instruments by which to measure views of the balance between length and quality of life (Mutran, Danis, Bratton, Sudha, & Hanson, 1997). These two scales are designed to measure the desire for life-sustaining treatment—Desire for Length of Benefit Scale (DLBS) to measure desire for treatment as a function of the duration of survival after treatment, and Desire for Probable Benefit Scale (DPBS) to measure desire for treatment as a function of the probability of success of treatment.

Scores for DLBS were derived by assigning a value of 1 to all affirmative responses and a value of 0 to all negative responses, and then summing these numbers. Scores range from 0 to 7. Scores for DPBS were derived from the average response to the three items and thus range from 0 to 100. Scores obtained through administration of the scales to patients with short life expectancy may be found in Danis et al. (1996).

Danis (1998) reports that the DPBS was at times difficult to administer because probability is a difficult concept for some people to understand. A few wanted to say 100% when they meant they always wanted the treatment even though there was very low probability of success (Danis, 1998).

PSYCHOMETRIC PROPERTIES

The instruments were administered by interview to 244 patients in one teaching hospital, with an age of at least 50 years and a short life expectancy due to end-stage heart, lung, or liver disease, metastatic cancer, or lymphoma. Cronbach's alpha for DLBS was .91, for DPBS .88. The relationship of these scales to the Desire to Prolong Life Scale was .48 for DLBS and .355 for DPBS (Mutran et al., 1997), providing some initial support for validity.

SUMMARY AND CRITIQUE

The study for which these instruments were developed focused on the degree to which patient preferences about the use of life-sustaining treatment were related to their actual use. The majority of these patients wanted to receive a life-sustaining treatment if it would prolong life for any length of time, and many were willing to have such a treatment even if it had no probability of working. Patient preferences were not related to life-sustaining treatment use.

Limited evidence assessing these instruments' validity could be located.

REFERENCES

Danis, M., Mutran, E., Garrett, J. M., Stearns, S. C., Slifkin, R. T., Hanson, L., Williams, J. F., & Churchill, L. R. (1996). A prospective study of the impact of patient preferences on life-sustaining treatment and hospital cost. *Critical Care Medicine, 24,* 1811-1817.

Danis, M. (1998). Letter to author.

Mutran, E. J., Danis, M., Bratton, K. A., Sudha, S., & Hanson, L. (1997). Attitudes of the critically ill toward prolonging life: The role of social support. *The Gerontologist, 37,* 192-199.

Instrument 2.4

DESIRE FOR PROBABLE BENEFIT SCALE

Before I ask you any more questions, I would like to give you some information about certain treatments that you may be familiar with.

Cardiopulmonary Resuscitation (CPR): If a person's heart stops beating, doctors can sometimes make it start again. They do this by pushing on the chest, forcing air into the lungs, giving medicines in the veins, and giving electrical shocks to the chest. The person is often on a breathing machine afterwards.

Breathing Machine: When a person's lungs fail, they may require a breathing machine. It pumps air in and out of the lungs through a tube that is inserted through the mouth or nose into the lungs, and does the work of breathing for a patient.

Intensive Care: As you may know when people become very sick, they are often cared for in an intensive care unit in order to watch them carefully. This is an area in the hospital where patients can receive special nursing attention, and monitoring of blood pressure and heart rhythm. Patients are monitored by being hooked up to machines and having tubes in blood vessels. They may be treated with medicines given by vein. They may use different treatments. For example, dialysis can be used for kidney failure, and breathing machines can be used if a patient's lungs stop working. It is hard to tell how well a person will do when he or she goes into the intensive care unit.

Now, I am going to ask you to complete some statements about the treatments that I have talked about (SHOW CUE CARD): Please use this card for your answers to the next 3 questions. It shows the chance of living from 0% to 100%, and all the numbers in between. At 0% there is no chance of living, at 50% the chance of living is the same as the chance of dying; at 100% a person is certain to live.

I would like you to tell me when you would be willing to have a treatment. As you answer this question, please think of your life as you currently live it. If you pick a point down here (POINT TO 0-10%) that would mean that you would want to have a treatment even when there is a small chance that the treatment will work. If you pick a point here (POINT TO 50%), this means you would be willing to have a treatment if the chances of the living or dying are the same. If you pick a point up here (POINT BETWEEN 90-100%) that would mean you would want the treatment only if it is extremely likely to work. If you would never want a treatment, regardless of how likely it is to work, you can tell me so. Now, I'd like you to complete this statement.

IF PATIENT NEVER WANTS LIFE-SUSTAINING TREATMENT, CHECK "NEVER"
AND CODE AS 100%.

1. Now, I'd like you to complete this statement:

   If my heart stopped beating, I would be willing to have my heart revived if
   the chance of surviving were at least:

   0%_____ 100% never_____
      0 10 20 30 40 50 60 70 80 90 100

   Could you tell me why you made this choice?_____
   _____

2. Now, I'd like you to complete this statement.

   If I were unable to breath on my own, I would be willing to go on a
   breathing machine if the chance of surviving were at least:

   0%_____ 100% never_____
      0 10 20 30 40 50 60 70 80 90 100

   Could you tell me why you made this choice?_____
   _____

3. Now, I would like you to complete this statement:

   If I were very sick, I would be willing to go into the intensive care unit if
   the chance of surviving were at least:

   0%_____ 100% never_____
      0 10 20 30 40 50 60 70 80 90 100

   Could you tell me why you made this choice?_____
   _____

DESIRE FOR LENGTH OF BENEFIT SCALE

Would you want to receive a life-sustaining treatment if it would prolong your
life for at least . . .

	No	Yes
5 years	0	1
2 years	0	1
1 year	0	1
6 months	0	1
3 months	0	1
1 month	0	1
1 week	0	1

SOURCE: Adapted from M. Danis and E. Mutran. Reprinted with permission.

LIFE SUPPORT PREFERENCES QUESTIONNAIRE (LSPQ)

Developed by Dawn K. Beland
and Robin D. Froman

INSTRUMENT DEVELOPMENT, ADMINISTRATION, AND SCORING

Although the Patient Self-Determination Act has legalized the importance of introducing life-support options, it is not yet clear how this subject is best presented to patients. The Life Support Preferences Questionnaire (LSPQ) was developed to facilitate such discussions by providing a mechanism for educating patients and their families about the array of life-support choices beyond the do not resuscitate (DNR) and mechanical ventilation options.

Item responses indicating a preference for life-support intervention were given a 1, preferences for withholding support a 0, and then summed for a total scale score of 0 to 6. High scores indicate preference for supportive interventions.

PSYCHOMETRIC PROPERTIES

The LSPQ is built on a prior scale authored by Zweibel and Cassel (1989), in which the vignettes were created by experts in biomedical ethics and geriatrics. Beland and Froman assumed and accepted the content validity of the earlier scale but added two vignettes more appropriate for a broader age range. These new vignettes deal with antibiotic use even when a person is in a persistent vegetative state and dialysis for an adolescent. The content domain of the LSPQ is "life-extending care."

Ten graduate nursing students and 5 nonhealth professionals reviewed the total item pool for clarity of presentation. Nurses, including a researcher, reviewed the vignettes for face validity and content sampling and agreed that the vignettes clearly posed questions about life support preferences, forced personal decision making, and included a variety of ages and illnesses (Beland & Froman, 1995).

The LSPQ was tested on a convenience sample of 116 healthy adults. Stability of responses 2 weeks apart ranged from 77% to 95% on the various items, with an average of 85%. Stability for the total scale score was .73. This evidence supports respondents' consistency of attitudes over a brief time. Factor analysis gave evidence of one dominant theme underlying the items, supporting the use of the total sum score as an estimate of life-support preference.

SUMMARY AND CRITIQUE

Beland and Froman caution that the LSPQ has thus far been used with healthy adults and not with hospitalized or soon-to-be-hospitalized populations. Although their responses provide initial evidence of reliability and unidimensional factorial validity, the profile of responses from healthy individuals could be expected to be different from those of an inpatient population (Beland & Froman, 1995).

Procedures by which content validity of the Zweibel and Cassel scale was established were not completely described in their original work (Zweibel & Cassel, 1989), leading to questions of whether its content validity should have been assumed. Created by a group of researchers expert in biomedical ethics and geriatrics, the vignettes represent scenarios of decisions about use of life-extending care required for an older patient unable to speak for himself or herself. The original set dealt with ventilation, resuscitation, chemotherapy, amputation, and tube feeding (Zweibel & Cassel, 1989). Many other clinical conditions likely would fall in this domain, and perhaps a more relevant definition of domain might relate to such decision characteristics as degree of certainty and potential consequences. Evidence of sensitivity of the LPSQ to intervention could not be located.

REFERENCES

Beland, D. K., & Froman, R. D. (1995). Preliminary validation of a measure of life support preferences. *Image, 27,* 307-310.

Zweibel, N. R., & Cassel, C. K. (1989). Treatment choices at the end of life: A comparison of decisions by older patients and their physician-selected proxies. *The Gerontologist, 29,* 615-621.

Instrument 2.5

LIFE SUPPORT PREFERENCES

Please review each case individually and choose the answer that best describes your preference for life-support. Please do not leave any blank responses and feel free to write in comments or explanations as appropriate.

Case #1

You recently suffered a major stroke leaving you in a coma and unable to breathe without a machine. After a few months, the doctor determines that it is unlikely that you will come out of the coma. If your doctor had asked whether to try to revive you if your heart stopped beating in this situation, what would you have told the doctor to do?

a. I would have told the doctor *to try* to revive my heart if it stopped beating knowing that the underlying condition would not have improved and may even have worsened it.

b. I would have the doctor *not to try* to revive my heart if it stopped beating.

Explain: _____

_____

Case #2

You are an elderly single person and have been in a persistent vegetative state with no hope for functional recovery. You are able to open your eyes and occasionally focus but have no recognition of friends and family. You are able to breathe on your own through a tube in your neck, and are artificially fed through a tube in your stomach. You recently developed pneumonia. The doctor tells your family that if the pneumonia is not treated with antibiotics, you will die. What would you want your family to tell the doctor to do?

a. I would want my family to tell the doctor *not to treat* the pneumonia with antibiotics and allow me to die.

b. I would want my family to tell the doctor *to treat* the pneumonia with antibiotics and allow me to continue in my present condition.

Explain: _____

_____

Case #3

You have been diagnosed as having a type of cancer that probably can not be cured. Your doctor indicates that chemotherapy (drug therapy) is available. The doctor explains that the chemotherapy may help you live longer. The doctor also tells you about the side effects of chemotherapy that can make you very ill. They can include severe nausea and vomiting, diarrhea, and hair loss. What would you decide to do?

a. I would decide *I did not want* chemotherapy knowing the length of my life might be shorter but that I would avoid the side effects of chemotherapy.

b. I would decide *I did want* chemotherapy knowing my life might be extended and that I might feel very ill.

Explain: _____

_____

Case #4

You are unable to make medical decisions for yourself because you have been declared mentally incompetent because of advanced Alzheimer's disease. You are a diabetic and have developed an untreatable infection in your leg. The doctor recommends to your family that unless you have your leg removed, you will die in a very short time. What would you have your family tell the doctor to do?

a. I would want my family to tell the doctor *to remove* the leg and allow me to continue in my present condition without the ability to walk.

b. I would want my family to tell the doctor *not to remove* the leg and allow me to die within a short time.

Explain: _____

_____

Case #5

You broke your hip and are recuperating from an operation to repair it. Since the operation you have had constant untreatable hip pain that may never change. You have become severely withdrawn due to your pain and will not speak to anyone. You refuse to eat and after several days the doctor wants to feed you using a feeding tube placed into your stomach. What would you have the doctor do?

a. I would *not want* the doctor to place a feeding tube into my stomach to feed me knowing that without nutrition the risk of other complications or death will increase.

b. I would *want* the doctor to place a feeding tube in my stomach despite my refusal knowing that I will have chronic hip pain.

Explain: _____

_____

Case #6

You have an adolescent relative who suffered trauma at birth and has had a poor quality of life since birth. Recently your relative developed kidney failure. The doctors tell your family that they may be able to keep your relative alive with the use of daily dialysis. Dialysis would require three hours of daily blood cleansing by a machine. If you were asked to make the decision, what would you want the doctors to do?

a. I would want the doctors *to use* dialysis to substitute kidney functioning knowing that the underlying birth defects and impairments would not improve.

b. I would want the doctors *not to use* dialysis and allow the adolescent to die.

Explain: _____

_____

SOURCE: From "Preliminary validation of a measure of life support preferences," by D. K. Beland and R. D. Froman, 1995, *Image, 27*, pp. 307-310. Reprinted with permission. LSPQ © D. Beland and R. Froman.

CARDIOPULMONARY RESUSCITATION PREFERENCE SCALE (CPR PREF)

Developed by Ronald S. Schonwetter,
Robert M. Walker, David R. Kramer,
and Bruce E. Robinson

INSTRUMENT DEVELOPMENT, ADMINISTRATION, AND SCORING

Patients' informed choices about cardiopulmonary resuscitation (CPR) should be a frequent occurrence and should include at a minimum the elements of informed consent—prognosis, risks and benefits of CPR, and alternatives. Schonwetter, Walker, Kramer, and Robinson (1993) have noted that past studies show physicians frequently do not discuss CPR with patients. Other work shows that information about the effects and outcomes of CPR might be an important determinant of patients' CPR choices, with those most informed more likely to reject it. Other work also shows that patients greatly overestimate their chances of surviving CPR and that the desire for it in hypothetical conditions of terminal disease was much stronger in people of lower rather than higher socioeconomic status (SES). The SES variables that define these groups may be proxy variables for underlying life values (Schonwetter, Walker, Kramer, & Robinson, 1994).

The Cardiopulmonary Resuscitation Preference Scale (CPR Pref) was administered by interview. Standard descriptions of cardiopulmonary arrest, CPR, and outcome data were provided with the five hypothetical scenarios. The interviewer used open-ended questions and prompts to assess the subjects' knowledge of the CPR procedure. The subjects were considered to understand these issues if they agreed it involved both mouth-to-mouth breathing and chest compressions. In some versions of the scale, participants recorded their preferences for each on a 5-point Likert-type scale: (a) definitely wanting CPR, (b) probably wanting CPR, (c) unsure, (d) probably not wanting CPR, and (e) definitely not wanting CPR. A summary index of overall desire for CPR was created by assigning a numeric value to three categories (desires CPR = 2, unsure = 1, declines CPR = 0) and summing. Additional questions were asked and may be obtained from the authors (Schonwetter et al., 1994).

PSYCHOMETRIC PROPERTIES

The CPR Pref was administered to 102 independent life-care community members more than 62 years of age, with high levels of education and of physical and mental health and 64 ambulatory patients from the Veterans Hospital Geriatric Clinic. Test-retest reliability with a group of 10 community-residing elderly people was .87. Approximately half of the participants from both settings desired CPR in the severe illness scenario, decreasing to approximately 20% in the three other scenarios.

This instrument has shown sensitivity to an educational intervention about CPR and its outcomes, with significant decreases in desire for CPR seen in three of the five scenarios (current state, hospitalization with severe illness, and terminal disease). CPR information was associated with changing preferences even among people with living wills (Walker, Schonwetter, Kramer, & Robinson, 1995). Survival estimates were more strongly associated with desire for CPR after the educational intervention. No control group was used in several of the studies (Schonwetter et al., 1993, 1994).

People with living wills were quite variable in their CPR preferences, indicating that one cannot reliably infer what an individual's preference might be by the mere fact that he or she has a living will, nor can one assume that those preferences are clear and certain (Schonwetter et al., 1995). Measures of life values showed a predictable relationship with CPR preference in the various scenarios, supporting validity of the scale (Schonwetter, Walker, Solomon, Indurkhya, & Robinson, 1996).

SUMMARY AND CRITIQUE

Because specific preferences regarding CPR were rarely recorded in the living wills of study participants who had them (Walker et al., 1995), specific indication of this preference would be useful. The CPR Pref offers this opportunity.

The CPR Pref has been used primarily in times of medical stability and thus likely does not reflect decisions that would actually be made at times of medical crisis or change in health status. In addition, responses to its hypothetical scenarios may not reflect decision making in real-life situations. Outcome data about CPR that were presented were general and might not be accurate for each specific clinical scenario (Schonwetter et al., 1993).

This instrument has primarily been used with highly educated white populations. Very little study of the validity of this instrument could be located, including justification of its content validity. The percentage of participants desiring CPR in each scenario was current condition 66%, acute illness 33%, terminal disease 8%, functional impairment 8%, and dementia 7% (Schonwetter et al., 1996).

Currency and completeness of the instrument as it appears following the references could not be verified with the authors.

REFERENCES

Schonwetter, R. S., Walker, R. M., Kramer, D. R., & Robinson, B. E. (1993). Resuscitation decision making in the elderly: The value of outcome data. *Journal of General Internal Medicine, 8,* 295-300.

Schonwetter, R. S., Walker, R. M., Kramer, D. R., & Robinson, B. E. (1994). Socioeconomic status and resuscitation preferences in the elderly. *Journal of Applied Gerontology, 13,* 157-171.

Schonwetter, R. S., Walker, R. M., Solomon, M., Indurkhya, A., & Robinson, B. E. (1996). Life values, resuscitation preferences and the applicability of living wills in an older population. *Journal of the American Geriatrics Society, 44,* 954-958.

Walker, R. M., Schonwetter, R. S., Kramer, D. R., & Robinson, B. E. (1995). Living wills and resuscitation preferences in an elderly population. *Archives of Internal Medicine, 155,* 171-175.

Instrument 2.6

STANDARD DESCRIPTION
OF CARDIOPULMONARY ARREST

"Cardiopulmonary arrest or sudden arrest is a term used when a person's heart or breathing stops for any reason, and that person does not get enough blood to the brain and other body parts to remain alive."

SOURCE: From "Socioeconomic status and resuscitation preferences in the elderly," by R. S. Schonwetter, R. M. Walker, D. R. Kramer, and B. E. Robinson, 1994, *Journal of Applied Gerontology, 13*, pp. 157-171. Reprinted with permission of Sage Publications, Inc.

Cardiopulmonary Resuscitation Information and Hypothetical Scenarios

A. Standard Description of Cardiopulmonary Resuscitation (CPR)

CPR involves a number of procedures that attempt to start the heart beating and maintain breathing and blood flow should someone's heart stop or breathing stop. CPR may involve mouth-to-mouth breathing or a breathing tube in the lungs and pressing on the chest or closed heart massage. It may also involve using special devices to deliver electricity and shock the heart to begin beating. It may involve giving medications into a person's veins or being hooked up to a breathing machine or mechanical ventilator.

B. Hypothetical Scenarios

1. *Current state of health:* If you were asked today to make a decision about whether or not you wanted CPR performed on you, what would you say?
   (a) yes   (b) no   (c) unsure

2. *Hospitalized with severe illness:* If you enter the hospital with a rapidly progressive severe illness requiring intensive and invasive treatment and the prognosis is unclear, would you want CPR?   (a) yes   (b) no   (c) unsure

3. *Terminal disease:* If you have a terminal disease like cancer and your life expectancy is less than 6 months no matter what type of medical treatment you receive, would you want CPR?   (a) yes   (b) no   (c) unsure

4. *Functional impairment, normal cognition:* If you have a major accident and are able to talk and understand what is going on but need to have someone else dress, bathe, feed, and move you and you could not control your bowels and urine—essentially, you are not able to do anything yourself and there is no chance of recovery, would you want CPR?
   (a) yes   (b) no   (c) unsure

5. *Cognitive impairment, normal physical state:* Imagine your mind is not what it used to be and you did not know your name, where you were, and did not recognize anyone around you. You would forget if you just ate or went to the

bathroom. Physically, however, you are in good shape, would you want CPR?
(a) yes   (b) no   (c) unsure

C. Descriptive Information About CPR and CPR Outcome Data

Descriptive information: Resuscitation may be successful by bringing a person back from almost death and start their heart and/or breathing as well as possibly bringing the person back to his or her original lifestyle. Resuscitation can be accompanied by many complications and injuries. Patients may end up on breathing machines forever, although this is rare. More commonly, they may have brain damage as a result of not getting enough oxygen to the brain. During the process, one may have broken ribs, a collapsed lung, broken teeth, a ruptured stomach, or burnt skin on the chest and these may cause severe pain to the patient if they survive. On the other hand, CPR may be the only thing to save someone's life.

Outcome Data: Recent studies on CPR in hospitalized patients of all ages have shown that attempts to restart the heart are successful less than half the time. In addition, one third of the patients older than 70 years who needed CPR had their heart restarted. These studies further showed that while less than half the patients had their heart and breathing restarted, less than two of 10 patients of all ages in whom CPR was attempted lived to leave the hospital alive. In addition, in patients older than 70 years, less than one of 10 lived to leave the hospital alive. Of those that left the hospital alive, most had disabilities that prevented a normal lifestyle.

SOURCE: From "Living wills and resuscitation preferences in an elderly population," by R. M. Walker, R. S. Schonwetter, D. R. Kramer, and B. E. Robinson, 1995, *Archives of Internal Medicine, 155,* pp. 171-175. Copyright 1995, American Medical Association. Reprinted with permission.

PREFERENCE OF LIFE-SUSTAINING TREATMENT QUESTIONNAIRE (PLSTQ)

Developed by Jiska Cohen-Mansfield,
Janet A. Droge, and Nathan Billig

INSTRUMENT DEVELOPMENT, ADMINISTRATION, AND SCORING

The Preference of Life-Sustaining Treatment Questionnaire (PLSTQ) was developed to study whether elderly hospitalized patients formed preferences regarding the use of specific medical treatments and the level of certainty with which these preferences were made. It assesses patients' preferences for or against nine treatment options: temporary or permanent tube feeding, resuscitation, temporary or permanent use of a respirator, amputation, kidney dialysis, radiation, chemotherapy, antibiotics, and blood transfusion. The preferences for each treatment are tested under three hypothetical conditions of future cognitive ability: intact (as you are now), permanently confused, and permanently unconscious. The preference is rated on a 7-point scale addressing direction and certainty of preference: 1 = absolutely does not want, 2 = no, 3 = uncertain but leaning toward a no, 4 = does not know, 5 = uncertain but leaning toward a yes, 6 = yes, and 7 = absolutely want the intervention. The PLSTQ does not provide details about the nature or outcomes of treatment. It is available in large print (Cohen-Mansfield, Droge, & Billig, 1992).

PSYCHOMETRIC PROPERTIES

The treatment options contained in the PLSTQ were selected on the basis of the literature as well as reports by geriatric physicians and nurses that indicated these are life-sustaining treatments around which decision making occurs most often in the hospital (content validity). Test-retest reliablity averaged .81. The instrument was tested with 97 elderly hospitalized patients (Cohen-Mansfield et al., 1992) and 103 nursing home residents (Cohen-Mansfield et al., 1991).

SUMMARY AND CRITIQUE

Among the hospitalized patients, 88% formed specific preferences for medical treatments and were certain about the decisions they were making. This suggests that it may be possible to make inferences regarding patient preferences for a particular treatment based on their preferences for other treatments. Studies of the predictive power of one scenario for another could clarify this issue. Two thirds of participants were less likely to want treatments under a condition of further cognitive functioning decline. One of the uses of the PLSTQ is to document these specific preferences by treatment and future cognitive condition.

A subgroup of patients characterized by depressive symptoms and low education was more likely not to have formed an opinion about treatments or to have a preference for receiving treatment most of the time. Among the nursing home residents, 41% manifested this pattern (Cohen-Mansfield et al., 1992). Evidence about the PLSTQ's sensitivity to interventions with this or other groups could not be located.

Thus far, the PLSTQ has primarily been tested with highly educated whites, and the nursing home residents were largely Jewish. This limits the generalizability of the findings.

REFERENCES

Cohen-Mansfield, J., Droge, J. A., & Billig, N. (1992). Factors influencing hospital patients' preferences in the utilization of life-sustaining treatments. *The Gerontologist, 32,* 89-95.

Cohen-Mansfield, J., Rabinovich, B. A., Lipson, S., Fein, A., Gerber, B., Weisman, S., & Pawlson, L. G. (1991). The decision to execute a durable power of attorney for health care and preferences regarding the utilization of life-sustaining treatments in nursing home residents. *Archives of Internal Medicine, 151,* 289-294.

Instrument 2.7

PREFERENCES FOR LIFE-SUSTAINING
TREATMENT QUESTIONNAIRE (PLSTQ)

Name_____ Unit_____

"I would now like to ask about your wishes in regard to some specific questions. These concern medical treatments that are used for some patients:"

[All conditions are assumed irreversible; however, other conditions are not assumed, i.e., nothing in addition to their current condition. Predictions of pain and quality of life are based totally on the above and are unknown otherwise. If patient has a detailed answer, like "it depends on . . ." try to find what it depends on and write it down on a separate sheet of paper.]

A. 1. If your heart stopped tomorrow, would you want to be resuscitated? How sure are you? Assume you are otherwise as you are now. [Explain resuscitate—restart heart]

1	2	3	4	5	6	7
absolutely does not want	no	uncertain but leaning towards a no	does not know	uncertain but leaning towards a yes	yes	absolutely want the intervention

(if 4) It depends on_____

2. If you ever became permanently confused and your heart stopped, would you want to be resuscitated? How sure are you? [Explain confused—if your mind or memory were not working properly]

1	2	3	4	5	6	7
absolutely does not want	no	uncertain but leaning towards a no	does not know	uncertain but leaning towards a yes	yes	absolutely want the intervention

(if 4) It depends on_____

3. If you were permanently in a coma and your heart stopped, would you want to be resuscitated? How sure are you?

1	2	3	4	5	6	7
absolutely does not want	no	uncertain but leaning towards a no	does not know	uncertain but leaning towards a yes	yes	absolutely want the intervention

(if 4) It depends on_____

B. 1. If you were temporarily unable to be fed by mouth, would you want to be tube fed? Assume you are otherwise as you are now. [Explain tube fed through gastrostomy]

1	2	3	4	5	6	7
absolutely does not want	no	uncertain but leaning towards a no	does not know	uncertain but leaning towards a yes	yes	absolutely want the intervention

(if 4) It depends on_____

2. If you were permanently confused and temporarily unable to be fed would you want to be tube fed?

1	2	3	4	5	6	7
absolutely does not want	no	uncertain but leaning towards a no	does not know	uncertain but leaning towards a yes	yes	absolutely want the intervention

(if 4) It depends on_____

3. If you were permanently in a coma and temporarily unable to be fed would you want to be tube fed?

1	2	3	4	5	6	7
absolutely does not want	no	uncertain but leaning towards a no	does not know	uncertain but leaning towards a yes	yes	absolutely want the intervention

(if 4) It depends on_____

C. 1. If you were permanently unable to be fed by mouth, would you want to be tube fed? Assume you are otherwise as you are now. [Explain tube fed through gastrostomy]

1	2	3	4	5	6	7
absolutely does not want	no	uncertain but leaning towards a no	does not know	uncertain but leaning towards a yes	yes	absolutely want the intervention

(if 4) It depends on_____

2. If you were permanently confused and permanently unable to be fed would you want to be tube fed?

1	2	3	4	5	6	7
absolutely does not want	no	uncertain but leaning towards a no	does not know	uncertain but leaning towards a yes	yes	absolutely want the intervention

(if 4) It depends on_____

3. If you were permanently in a coma and permanently unable to be fed would you want to be tube fed?

1	2	3	4	5	6	7
absolutely does not want	no	uncertain but leaning towards a no	does not know	uncertain but leaning towards a yes	yes	absolutely want the intervention

(if 4) It depends on_____

D. 1. If you had an infection in your foot and the only way to stop it from spreading was to amputate, would you want to undergo the amputation? Assume that you are otherwise as you are now.

1	2	3	4	5	6	7
absolutely does not want	no	uncertain but leaning towards a no	does not know	uncertain but leaning towards a yes	yes	absolutely want the intervention

(if 4) It depends on_____

2. If you were permanently confused and had an infection in your foot and the only way to stop it was to amputate, would you want to undergo the amputation?

1	2	3	4	5	6	7
absolutely does not want	no	uncertain but leaning towards a no	does not know	uncertain but leaning towards a yes	yes	absolutely want the intervention

(if 4) It depends on_____

3. If you were permanently in a coma and had an infection in your foot and the only way to stop it was to amputate, would you want to undergo the amputation?

1	2	3	4	5	6	7
absolutely does not want	no	uncertain but leaning towards a no	does not know	uncertain but leaning towards a yes	yes	absolutely want the intervention

(if 4) It depends on_____

E. 1. If you became temporarily unable to breathe on your own, would you want to be placed on a respirator? Assume that you are otherwise as you are now.

1	2	3	4	5	6	7
absolutely does not want	no	uncertain but leaning towards a no	does not know	uncertain but leaning towards a yes	yes	absolutely want the intervention

(if 4) It depends on_____

2. If you were permanently confused and became temporarily unable to breathe on your own, would you want to be placed on a respirator?

1	2	3	4	5	6	7
absolutely does not want	no	uncertain but leaning towards a no	does not know	uncertain but leaning towards a yes	yes	absolutely want the intervention

(if 4) It depends on_____

3. If you were permanently in a coma and became temporarily unable to breathe on your own, would you want to be placed on a respirator?

1	2	3	4	5	6	7
absolutely does not want	no	uncertain but leaning towards a no	does not know	uncertain but leaning towards a yes	yes	absolutely want the intervention

(if 4) It depends on_____

F. 1. If your kidneys failed, would you want kidney dialysis? Assume that you are otherwise as you are now.

1	2	3	4	5	6	7
absolutely does not want	no	uncertain but leaning towards a no	does not know	uncertain but leaning towards a yes	yes	absolutely want the intervention

(if 4) It depends on_____

2. If you were permanently confused and your kidneys failed, would you want kidney dialysis?

1	2	3	4	5	6	7
absolutely does not want	no	uncertain but leaning towards a no	does not know	uncertain but leaning towards a yes	yes	absolutely want the intervention

(if 4) It depends on_____

3. If you were permanently in a coma and your kidneys failed, would you want kidney dialysis?

1	2	3	4	5	6	7
absolutely does not want	no	uncertain but leaning towards a no	does not know	uncertain but leaning towards a yes	yes	absolutely want the intervention

(if 4) It depends on_____

G. 1. If you got pneumonia, would you want to be treated with antibiotics? Assume that you are otherwise as you are now.

1	2	3	4	5	6	7
absolutely does not want	no	uncertain but leaning towards a no	does not know	uncertain but leaning towards a yes	yes	absolutely want the intervention

(if 4) It depends on_____

2. If you ever became permanently confused and got pneumonia, would you want to be treated with antibiotics?

1	2	3	4	5	6	7
absolutely does not want	no	uncertain but leaning towards a no	does not know	uncertain but leaning towards a yes	yes	absolutely want the intervention

(if 4) It depends on_____

3. If you were permanently in a coma and got pneumonia, would you want to be treated with antibiotics?

1	2	3	4	5	6	7
absolutely does not want	no	uncertain but leaning towards a no	does not know	uncertain but leaning towards a yes	yes	absolutely want the intervention

(if 4) It depends on_____

H. 1. If you got cancer, would you want to be treated with radiation therapy? Assume that you are otherwise as you are now.

1	2	3	4	5	6	7
absolutely does not want	no	uncertain but leaning towards a no	does not know	uncertain but leaning towards a yes	yes	absolutely want the intervention

(if 4) It depends on_____

2. If you were permanently confused and you got cancer, would you want to be treated with radiation therapy?

1	2	3	4	5	6	7
absolutely does not want	no	uncertain but leaning towards a no	does not know	uncertain but leaning towards a yes	yes	absolutely want the intervention

(if 4) It depends on_____

3. If you were permanently in a coma and you got cancer, would you want to be treated with radiation therapy?

1	2	3	4	5	6	7
absolutely does not want	no	uncertain but leaning towards a no	does not know	uncertain but leaning towards a yes	yes	absolutely want the intervention

(if 4) It depends on_____

I. 1. If you got cancer, would you want to be treated with chemotherapy? Assume that you are otherwise as you are now.

1	2	3	4	5	6	7
absolutely does not want	no	uncertain but leaning towards a no	does not know	uncertain but leaning towards a yes	yes	absolutely want the intervention

(if 4) It depends on_____

2. If you were permanently confused and you got cancer, would you want to be treated with chemotherapy?

1	2	3	4	5	6	7
absolutely does not want	no	uncertain but leaning towards a no	does not know	uncertain but leaning towards a yes	yes	absolutely want the intervention

(if 4) It depends on_____

3. If you were permanently in a coma and you got cancer, would you want to be treated with chemotherapy?

1	2	3	4	5	6	7
absolutely does not want	no	uncertain but leaning towards a no	does not know	uncertain but leaning towards a yes	yes	absolutely want the intervention

(if 4) It depends on_____

J. 1. If your blood count dropped sufficiently to threaten your life, would you want a blood transfusion? Assume that you are otherwise as you are now.

1	2	3	4	5	6	7
absolutely does not want	no	uncertain but leaning towards a no	does not know	uncertain but leaning towards a yes	yes	absolutely want the intervention

(if 4) It depends on_____

2. If you were permanently confused and your blood count dropped
   sufficiently to threaten your life, would you want a blood transfusion?

1	2	3	4	5	6	7
absolutely does not want	no	uncertain but leaning towards a no	does not know	uncertain but leaning towards a yes	yes	absolutely want the intervention

(if 4) It depends on_____

3. If you were permanently in a coma and your blood count dropped
   sufficiently to threaten your life, would you want a blood transfusion?

1	2	3	4	5	6	7
absolutely does not want	no	uncertain but leaning towards a no	does not know	uncertain but leaning towards a yes	yes	absolutely want the intervention

(if 4) It depends on_____

K. 1. If you became permanently unable to breathe on your own, would you
      want to be placed on a respirator? Assume that you are otherwise as
      you are now.

1	2	3	4	5	6	7
absolutely does not want	no	uncertain but leaning towards a no	does not know	uncertain but leaning towards a yes	yes	absolutely want the intervention

(if 4) It depends on_____

2. If you were permanently confused and became permanently unable to
   breathe on your own, would you want to be placed on a respirator?

1	2	3	4	5	6	7
absolutely does not want	no	uncertain but leaning towards a no	does not know	uncertain but leaning towards a yes	yes	absolutely want the intervention

(if 4) It depends on_____

3. If you were permanently in a coma and became permanently unable to
   breathe on your own, would you want to be placed on a respirator?

1	2	3	4	5	6	7
absolutely does not want	no	uncertain but leaning towards a no	does not know	uncertain but leaning towards a yes	yes	absolutely want the intervention

(if 4) It depends on_____

L. 1. If your condition deteriorated, would you like to be sent to the hospital? Assume that you are otherwise as you are now.

1	2	3	4	5	6	7
absolutely does not want	no	uncertain but leaning towards a no	does not know	uncertain but leaning towards a yes	yes	absolutely want the intervention

(if 4) It depends on_____

2. If you were permanently confused and your condition deteriorated, would you like to be sent to the hospital?

1	2	3	4	5	6	7
absolutely does not want	no	uncertain but leaning towards a no	does not know	uncertain but leaning towards a yes	yes	absolutely want the intervention

(if 4) It depends on_____

3. If you were permanently in a coma and your condition deteriorated, would you like to be sent to the hospital?

1	2	3	4	5	6	7
absolutely does not want	no	uncertain but leaning towards a no	does not know	uncertain but leaning towards a yes	yes	absolutely want the intervention

(if 4) It depends on_____

3 Patient Comprehension

A basic element to expression of a preference and to informed consent is sufficient understanding of the choices, including the level of uncertainty. Whereas most legal discussions of informed consent emphasize the amount and kind of information the professional provides, there is an ethical obligation to make reasonable efforts to assure patient comprehension. Little is known about how well this ethical obligation is implemented in common clinical and research settings. The instruments in this section provide a way to assess and document this understanding.

Formal assessment should address common patient misunderstandings particularly of risks and benefits associated with various treatments. Either risks or benefits may be inflated as a result of anxiety. For example, studies of prenatal genetic counseling have shown that most individuals perceive their risks in binary form (I either will or will not deliver a healthy baby) and that probability information about genetic inheritance has a limited impact on risk perception. Different ethnic groups may perceive risks and benefits quite differently. Furthermore, knowledge alone is not likely to be sufficient to assist individuals with a reasoned evaluation of the positive and negative consequences of alternate choices (Lerman et al., 1997).

Instruments assessing patient comprehension are essential. These outcome measures test various methods for helping patients understand complex information necessary to participate in decision making about testing and treatment, frequently in life-threatening situations.

Informed consent to participate in research is highly prescribed and is detailed in the review of the Deaconess Informed Consent Comprehension Test (which follows later in this chapter) as well as more completely in many other sources including Brody (1998). Research often involves an additional set of misconceptions, for example, the incorrect inference that procedures will be of immediate benefit to the participants themselves (therapeutic misconception), or participants not understanding that they could be receiving placebos.

It is common to find patients unable to recall significant information believed to be necessary to informed consent. The central question is whether legal and ethical standards will more consistently require evidence of patient understanding.

REFERENCES

Brody, B. A. (1998). *The ethics of biomedical research.* New York: Oxford University Press.
Lerman, C., Biesecker, B., Benkendorf, J. L., Kerner, J., Gomez-Caminero, A., Hughes, C., & Reed, M. M. (1997). Controlled trial of pretest education approaches to enhance informed decision-making for BRCA1 gene testing. *Journal of the National Cancer Institute, 89,* 148-157.

PRE-VIGNETTE KNOWLEDGE TEST
POST-VIGNETTE
COMPREHENSION TEST

Developed by Michele D. Krynski, Alexander J. Tymchuk,
and Joseph G. Ouslander

INSTRUMENT DEVELOPMENT, ADMINISTRATION, AND SCORING

Elderly people in long-term care facilities frequently have an incomplete understanding about various medical procedures including enteral feeding; yet, a decision about this treatment may well be a part of advance directive (AD) planning. Because existing data suggest that enteral feeding probably does not significantly prolong life, it is important that elders understand the risks and the benefits of this treatment.

The Pre-Vignette Knowledge Test and Post-Vignette Comprehension Test are given in response to a vignette in illustrated storybook format written at a fifth-grade level. The pretest, with a total score of 17 (mean score in the tested population was 10.5), is administered before presentation of the vignette, and the posttest, with a total score of 28 (mean score 22.8), after the vignette (Krynski, Tymchuk, & Ouslander, 1994).

PSYCHOMETRIC PROPERTIES

These instruments were pilot tested and then administered to 34 residential and 34 community-dwelling elders who were independent in activities of daily living, free of severe cognitive deficits, and who volunteered. Most had one or more stable chronic health problems. A geriatrician reviewed various presentations of information and illustrations including the content and order to ensure accuracy. Presumably, the pre- and posttests tested the same information.

Both community-dwelling and residential participants showed significant improvement in comprehension from initial to posttesting, with the former group showing significantly more improvement. This finding indicates sensitivity of the scale to intervention. The Mini-Mental State Examination was found to be the most useful instrument for prediction of comprehension, as were higher depression scores and lower social support. These findings are consistent with what theory would predict and therefore supportive of construct validity (Krynski et al., 1994).

SUMMARY AND CRITIQUE

Other than the geriatrician's review of content of the vignettes, no formal assessment of content validity could be located. Ouslander, Tymchuk, and Krynski note that a more direct measure of the quality and content of decision making would be helpful although they know of no such measure.

The instruments have been tested with a sample limited in size and more independent and cognitively intact than many people who might be faced with decisions about feeding tubes. In addition, the intervention depicted only one scenario, although the authors believe it contained the most common circumstances in which the decision to insert and withhold an enteral feeding tube would be made. These instruments also appear not to have been tested to determine their sensitivity to a range of intervention approaches.

REFERENCES

Krynski, M. D., Tymchuk, A. J., & Ouslander, J. G. (1994). How informed can consent be? New light on comprehension among elderly people making decisions about enteral tube feeding. *The Gerontologist, 34*, 36-43.

Ouslander, J. G., Tymchuk, A. J., & Krynski, M. D. (1993). Decisions about enteral tube feeding among the elderly. *Journal of the American Geriatrics Society, 41*, 70-77.

Instrument 3.1

SESSION ONE

NAME: _____

INTERVIEWER: _____

DATE: _____

PRE-VIGNETTE COMPREHENSION TEST

A Recent Jewish Home of the Aging policy requires that we ask you about what you would want the Jewish Home to do if you were very sick, not able to eat well, not able to speak your wishes clearly, and a specific medical treatment (enteral tube feeding) was available to you. We want to know if, after teaching you certain facts, you would or would not want this medical treatment.

Today, we are going to present a story about the enteral feeding tube. Before I read the story to you, I will ask you to complete a short true-false test to see how much you already know about the feeding tube. After the story, I will be asking you to complete a similar test.

Now I am going to ask you some questions regarding enteral feeding. In this part of the study, we are trying to find out what you already know about tube feeding through the stomach. Most of you probably know little or nothing about it, and that is fine. We are interested in people with many different backgrounds. It is all right if you want to guess at some of the questions because we don't expect you to know a lot about this subject. In fact, I would prefer that you guess the answers to the questions rather than leave anything blank. Right now I won't be able to tell you the answers to the questions, but we can talk about them at a later time if you like.

As we read these questions together, please mark true or false (T or F) beside every question. I would like you to mark true or false even if you are unsure of your answers. Please don't forget to put your name at the top of the first page.

CONDITION OF PATIENT

_____ 1. A patient is given a feeding tube when she cannot eat well.
_____ 2. A patient is given a feeding tube *only* when she cannot eat *anything* at all.
_____ 3. A patient is usually given a feeding tube when she has a disease which creates a serious eating problem for her.

ENTERAL FEEDING TUBE

_____ 4. A patient is given a feeding tube even when her eating problem will get better by itself without medical treatment.

_____ 5. Patients who can be helped by feeding tubes often are so sick that their mental and physical condition continues to get worse despite the tube.

_____ 6. Patients who can be helped by the feeding tube are in danger of getting many sores on their skin if they do not get medical treatment.

_____ 7. The best life-saving treatment for an ill patient who has serious trouble eating is to have someone spoon-feed the patient for the rest of her life.

_____ 8. The best life-saving treatment for an ill patient who has serious trouble eating is to have a feeding tube put into her stomach.

_____ 9. With the feeding tube in such a patient's stomach, the patient would probably not get enough food so as to starve to death.

_____ 10. A feeding tube in such a patient's stomach would probably not help her live longer.

_____ 11. In order for a patient to have the feeding tube in her stomach, she would have to undergo a small operation.

_____ 12. A feeding tube could cause such a patient to get more infections than she would have by having someone else spoon-feed her.

_____ 13. A feeding tube might cause a patient to have diarrhea.

_____ 14. At first, a patient might not be comfortable with the tube in her stomach, but she could probably get used to it.

_____ 15. A feeding tube could only help a serious feeding problem, but it could not cure a major disease.

_____ 16. Having a feeding tube would make sure than an ill patient did not get pneumonia.

_____ 17. A patient with a serious eating problem could choose to be spoon-fed by someone else.

_____ 18. If such a patient were spoon-fed by someone, she probably would get all the food her body needs.

_____ 19. No operation is needed in order for a patient to have the feeding tube put in her stomach.

_____ 20. A feeding tube operation is a common procedure known to many doctors.

_____ 21. Such an ill patient might get more sores on her skin if she were spoon-fed by someone else than if she had a feeding tube in her stomach.

_____ 22. If such a patient were spoon-fed by someone else, she would probably die in a few weeks or months anyway, because of (due to) her serious disease.

SOURCE: A. J. Tymchuk, J. G. Ouslander, M. D. Krynski, and Osterweil. Reprinted with permission.

Instrument 3.2

AN ILLUSTRATED VIGNETTE DEPICTING TUBE FEEDING

Alexander J. Tymchuk, Ph.D., and Joseph Ouslander, M.D., UCLA
© 1990, Drs. Tymchuk and Ouslander.

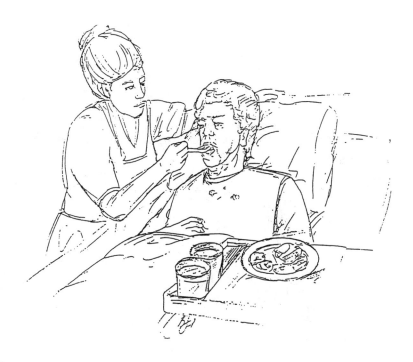

THE PROBLEM:

Let's think for a minute that you can no longer eat all the food your body
needs. From now on, you will need someone to feed you—either by hand or
through a feeding tube. You can't eat well because you have a serious disease. This disease is making you lose more and more of your mental and
physical abilities. Right now you can't even walk anymore. You can still recognize people and talk to them.

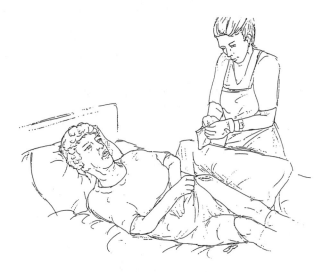

If you don't get enough food, you will become very weak. You could get sores on your skin because you are weak. You could also get infections that might make you very sick or even kill you.

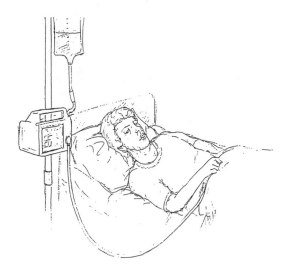

THE BEST LIFE-SAVING TREATMENT:

The best life-saving treatment for your problem with eating would be to have a feeding tube put into your stomach. Then you could be fed food through the tube.

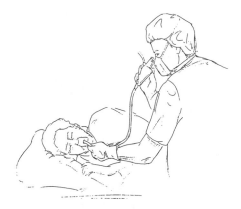

In order to have the tube, you would need a small operation. You would be given pain medicine to make you comfortable. The doctor would put a tube that acts like a telescope through your mouth and into your stomach. Then the doctor would use this tube that acts like a telescope to put a feeding tube through your abdomen and right into your stomach. Next, the tube that acts like a telescope would be taken out of your mouth. This operation has been done often.

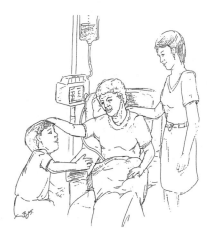

THE GOOD THINGS ABOUT THE FEEDING TUBE:

With a feeding tube, you could probably get all the food and fluids your body needs. You would probably live longer than if you didn't have the tube. This way you might not get sores on your skin or infections.

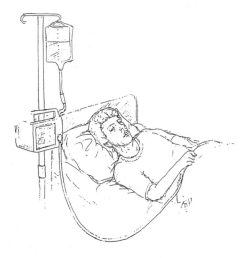

The tube from your abdomen into your stomach would stay there so you could be fed through it.

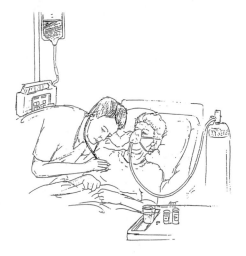

THE BAD THINGS ABOUT THE FEEDING TUBE:

Some bad things might happen as well. You might get more diarrhea (loose stool) by being fed through the tube. You could also get pneumonia from food getting into your lungs. You could die from pneumonia. You might get pneumonia even *without* the feeding tube, because of the disease that is making you unable to eat well.

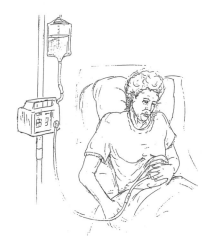

The tube would always be in your stomach. It might be uncomfortable at first—but you would probably get used to it. However, the feeding tube would not make your serious disease any better. You would still keep losing more and more of your mental and physical abilities.

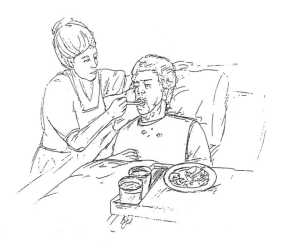

AN ALTERNATIVE WAY TO BE FED:

You might not want the feeding tube. Instead, you could be fed by someone else. However, this way you might not be able to get all the food and fluids your body needs due to the serious disease you have. If you did not get enough food, you might develop infections or sores on your skin.

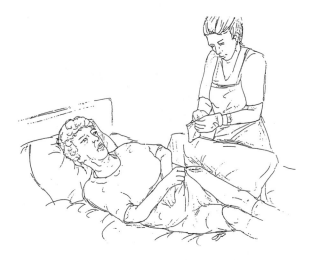

Even if you did get enough food by someone else feeding you, you could still get sores on your skin or infections because your body would still get much weaker.

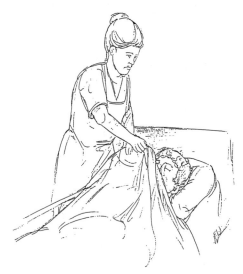

Without the feeding tube, you would probably die in a few weeks or months because your body would not get enough food. The decision to have or not have a feeding tube may be difficult to decide. You may want to discuss it with your doctor, social worker, religious leader, and family before making the decision.

ENTERAL TUBE FEEDING

THE PROBLEM:

Let's suppose for a minute that you can no longer eat all the food your body needs. From now on, you will need someone to feed you—either by hand or through a feeding tube. You can't eat well because you have a serious disease. This disease is making you lose more and more of your mental and physical abilities. Right now you can't even walk anymore. You can still recognize people and talk to them.

If you can't get enough food, you will become weak. You could get sores on your skin because you are weak. You could also get infections that might make you very sick or even kill you.

THE BEST LIFE-SAVING TREATMENT:

The best life-saving treatment for your problem with eating would be to have a feeding tube put into your stomach. Then you could be fed food through the tube.

In order to have the tube, you would need a small operation. You would be given pain medicine to make you comfortable. The doctor would put a tube that acts like a telescope through your mouth and into your stomach. Then the doctor would use this tube that acts like a telescope to put a feeding tube through your abdomen and right into your stomach. Next, the tube that acts like a telescope would be taken out of your mouth. This operation has been done often.

The tube from your abdomen into your stomach would stay there so you could be fed through it.

THE GOOD THINGS ABOUT THE FEEDING TUBE:

With a feeding tube, you could probably get all the food and fluids your body needs. You would probably live longer than if you didn't have the tube. This way you might not get sores on your skin or infections.

THE BAD THINGS ABOUT THE FEEDING TUBE:

Some bad things might happen as well. You might get more diarrhea (loose stool) by being fed through the tube. You could also get pneumonia from food getting into your lungs. You could die from pneumonia. You might get pneumonia even *without* the feeding tube, because of the disease that is making you unable to eat.

The tube would always be in your stomach. It might be uncomfortable at first—but you would probably get used to it. However, the feeding tube would not make your serious disease better. You would still keep losing more and more of your mental and physical abilities.

AN ALTERNATIVE WAY TO BE FED:

You might not want the feeding tube. Instead, you could be fed by someone else. However, this way you might not be able to get all the food and fluids your body needs due to the serious disease you have. If you did not get enough food, you might develop infections or sores on your skin.

Even if you get enough food by someone else feeding you, you could still get sores on your skin or infections because your body would still get weaker.

Without the feeding tube, you would probably die in a few weeks or months because your body would not get enough food. The decision to have or not have a feeding tube may be difficult to decide. You may want to discuss it with your doctor, social worker, religious leader, and family before making the decision.

Drs. Tymchuk, Ouslander,
Krynski, Osterweil

SOURCE: A. J. Tymchuk, J. G. Ouslander, M. D. Krynski, and Osterweil. Reprinted with permission.

Instrument 3.3

SESSION

NAME: _____
INTERVIEWER: _____
DATE: _____

POST-VIGNETTE COMPREHENSION TEST

Introduction (Interviewer reads aloud): We want to find out if we have been able to teach you some of the facts about enteral feeding. Right now, I just want you to answer true-false questions based on what the story says. At another time soon, your social worker or I will ask you to answer questions about what personal decisions you would make if you were in this situation. As we read these questions together, please mark true or false (T or F) beside every question. I would like you to mark true or false even if you are unsure of your answers. Please don't forget to put your name at the top of the first page.

CONDITION OF PATIENT

_____ 1. In this story, the patient is eating well.
_____ 2. In this story, the patient cannot eat at all.
_____ 3. In this story, the patient has a disease which creates a serious eating problem for her.
_____ 4. In this story, the patient's eating problem will get better by itself without medical treatment.
_____ 5. In this story, the patient could get many sores on her skin if she does not get medical treatment.
_____ 6. In this story, the patient cannot walk anymore.
_____ 7. In this story, the patient can no longer talk to her friends because of her main serious disease.

ENTERAL FEEDING TUBE

_____ 8. According to this story, the best life-saving treatment is to have someone spoon-feed the patient from now on.
_____ 9. According to this story, the best life-saving treatment is to have a feeding tube put into the patient's stomach.
_____ 10. According to the story, with the feeding tube in the patient's stomach, the patient would probably get enough food.
_____ 11. According to the story, the feeding tube would probably not help the patient live longer.

_____ 12. According to the story, the feeding tube could cause the patient to get more infections.

_____ 13. According to the story, the patient might get diarrhea from being fed through a feeding tube in her stomach.

_____ 14. According to the story, at first the patient might not be comfortable with the tube in her stomach, but she could probably get used to it.

_____ 15. According to the story, having a feeding tube put in her stomach would cure the patient's main disease.

_____ 16. According to the story, having a feeding tube would make sure that the patient did not get pneumonia.

_____ 17. According to the story, the patient could choose to be spoon-fed by someone else.

_____ 18. According to the story, if the patient were spoon-fed by someone, she would probably get all the food her body needs.

_____ 19. According to the story, the patient would have to have a small operation in order to have the feeding tube put in her stomach.

_____ 20. According to the story, the feeding tube operation is a common procedure known to many doctors.

_____ 21. The patient could get more sores on her skin if she were spoon-fed by someone else than if she had a feeding tube in her stomach.

_____ 22. If the patient were spoon-fed by someone else, she would probably die in a few weeks or months anyway because of (due to) her serious disease.

_____ 23. It is difficult to make the decision to have or not have a feeding tube. In the story, who are the persons mentioned who might be helpful in discussing the decision? Please check all persons you remember who were mentioned in the story.

        a. _____ family
        b. _____ social worker
        c. _____ religious leader (example: rabbi)
        d. _____ doctor
        e. _____ friends
        f. _____ lawyer
        g. _____ other

Drs. Tymchuk, Ouslander, Krynski, Osterweil

SOURCE: A. J. Tymchuk, J. G. Ouslander, M. D. Krynski, and Osterweil. Reprinted with permission.

Instrument 3.4

Name: _____

Interviewer: _____

Date: _____

POST-VIGNETTE STRUCTURED QUESTIONNAIRE

Introduction (Interviewer reads it aloud): Within the last few days, you attended a meeting in which you learned some facts about enteral tube feeding. Now I would like to ask you questions about what you would do if you had to make decisions about enteral tube feeding:

1. What would you want the Jewish Homes for the Aging to do if you were seriously ill and it had to be decided whether or not to give you a feeding tube in your stomach?

   _____
   _____
   _____

   Decision to have the feeding tube:

   ___ yes

   ___ no

2. Why did you make that choice?

   _____
   _____
   _____

3. What reasons were most important to you in making your choice?

   _____
   _____
   _____

4. Did any of these factors influence your decision?

   ___ Quality of life

   ___ Preventing other people from being negatively affected

   ___ Want to live as long as possible

   ___ Religious reasons

   ___ Don't want discomfort or pain

   ___ Don't want dependency because feels shameful

   ___ Want to live longer

   ___ Want to die quicker

   ___ Want to show care for significant others

   ___ Have lived long enough

   ___ Don't want to be a burden

   ___ Other _____

5. Is there anyone you would have liked to talk to before making up your mind to have or not have the feeding tube? (indicate relationship)
   Person: _____

6. In addition to the facts in the story, what other information would you have liked to have had before making your decision to have or not have the feeding tube?

   _____

   _____

   a.) Would you have liked more information about the stomach feeding tube?
      ___ yes
      ___ no
   b.) Would you have liked more information about the stomach feeding tube operation?
      ___ yes
      ___ no
   c.) Would you have like more information about the effects of being spoon-fed by another person?
      ___ yes
      ___ no

The interviewer reads aloud the following as she shows the subject the decision-making scales, with ratings from "Very Good" to "Very Bad": Now I would like to ask you a few questions about how you feel about our talk today. This is important because we want to find out how other people might feel about discussing issues like this one with their doctors.

7. How does our talk today make you feel?
   ___ Very Good
   ___ Neither Good Nor Bad
   ___ Very Bad

8. Does our talk make you worry about your health?
   ___ A Lot
   ___ Somewhat
   ___ Not At All

9. Do you think it is a good idea to talk about situations like this with your doctor before they happen so your doctor will know how you feel about them?
   ___ Very Good
   ___ Neither Good Nor Bad
   ___ Very Bad

10. a.) Would you want your doctor to ask you about this subject while you are as healthy as you are and don't need help to eat well?
    ___ Definitely Yes
    ___ Don't Care
    ___ Definitely No

Drs. Tymchuk, Ouslander, Krynski, Osterweil
SOURCE: A. J. Tymchuk, J. G. Ouslander, M. D. Krynski, and Osterweil. Reprinted with permission.

Instrument 3.5

RESIDENT'S NAME:_____

Your relative will be asked by the Jewish Home for the Aging to make a durable power of attorney decision about enteral tube feeding. Currently, the Jewish Home is required to obtain the stated wishes of all residents as to whether they would want the home to give them an enteral feeding tube should they become seriously ill and need the tube to survive—yet be unable to state their wishes. Soon your relative may be shown the enclosed vignette and may be asked to sign the Durable Power of Attorney Addendum. Please complete this form and mail it in the enclosed envelope.

1) Do you think your relative will sign under the *YES* or *NO* categories in the Durable Power of Attorney Addendum?

_____ I think *my relative* will say *YES* (accept enteral tube feeding).

_____ I think *my relative* will say *NO* (refuse enteral tube feeding).

2) Do *you* think your relative should say *YES* or *NO*?

_____ I think my relative should say *YES*.

_____ I think my relative should say *NO*.

3) How would you rate your relative's capacity to make a good decision?

_____ *Very good:* can express a choice which *would* be based on a reasonable weighing of the risks and benefits *and* a full consideration of all the information and consequences.

_____ *Good:* can indicate a choice based on a reasonable weighing of the risks and benefits, *but* it would *not* be with full consideration of all the potential consequences.

_____ *Fair:* can indicate a choice, but the choice would not be based on an understanding of the relevant information.

_____ *Poor:* is not able to make a decision or show a preference.

4) Have you spoken to your relative about this decision?

_____ Yes, we have spoken specifically about enteral tube feeding.

_____ We have spoken about life-sustaining measures *in general*, but not enteral tube feeding specifically.

_____ No, we have not spoken about these types of decisions.

5) How are you related to your relative? (Please indicate relationship)

THANK YOU FOR COMPLETING THIS FORM
Please return to Dr._____at the Jewish Home
Medical Department in the enclosed envelope.

ADDENDUM TO DURABLE POWER OF ATTORNEY FOR HEALTH CARE DECISIONS

ENTERAL FEEDING TUBE

Name: _____

I understand that the Jewish Home for the Aging *does* provide enteral tube feeding for *all* residents who become seriously ill and need the tube to survive—*unless* they refuse it.

In the event that I should become incapable of stating my wishes, I want the Jewish Home for the Aging to follow my wishes as stated in this document.

Enteral Feeding Tube Decision

Please sign under *YES* OR *NO*

YES: Should I become seriously ill and need the enteral feeding tube to survive—yet be unable to state my wishes, I want the Jewish Home for the Aging to provide the feeding tube for me.

_____
SIGNATURE

_____
DATE

_____
WITNESS

NO: Should I become seriously ill and need the enteral feeding tube to survive—yet be unable to state my wishes, I *do not* want the Jewish Home for the Aging to provide the feeding tube for me.

_____
SIGNATURE

_____
DATE

_____
WITNESS

SOURCE: A. J. Tymchuk, J. G. Ouslander, M. D. Krynski, and Osterweil. Reprinted with permission.

KNOWLEDGE ABOUT BREAST CANCER GENETICS AND BRCA1 TESTING PERCEPTIONS OF THE BENEFITS, LIMITATIONS, AND RISKS OF BRCA1 TESTING

Developed by Caryn Lerman, Steven Narod,
Kevin Schulman, Charita Hughes, Andres Gomez-Caminero,
George Bonney, Karen Gold, Bruce Trock, David Main,
Jane Lynch, Cecil Fulmore, Carrie Snyder, Stephen J. Lemon,
Theresa Conway, Patricia Tonin, Gilbert Lenoir, and Henry Lynch

INSTRUMENT DEVELOPMENT, ADMINISTRATION, AND SCORING

It is estimated that approximately 5% to 10% of all breast and ovarian cancers are attributable to one or more susceptibility genes that are inherited in an autosomal dominant fashion (Lerman, Daly, Masny, & Balshem, 1994). In response to the isolation of a breast-ovarian cancer susceptibility gene, BRCA1, biotechnology companies are already marketing genetic tests to health care providers and to the public (Lerman et al., 1997). The BRCA1 gene is highly penetrant, producing a risk of breast cancer that approaches 80% to 90% by age 70 (Lerman, Seay, Balshem, & Audrain, 1995). Because it is estimated that BRCA1 is the most prevalent gene for which genetic testing is available, the demand for testing among women with an affected first-degree relative is expected to be great. Male mutation carriers are at increased risk for prostate and colon cancer and can also transmit breast-ovarian cancer susceptibility to their daughters (Lerman et al., 1996).

For those patients who decide to be tested, medical and psychological management of the possible negative psychological sequelae will be important. Negative results from testing may also not be without psychological costs of worry and feelings of guilt. The documented inflated sense of personal risk, common in women, about these cancers underscores the need to educate them about complex aspects of genetics to ensure that their decisions about genetic testing are informed by knowledge rather than driven by anxiety. They need to understand the limitations and potential risks of genetic information, that genetic information is probabilistic, and the limitations of current options for breast and ovarian cancer prevention and early detection include the risk of genetic discrimination (Lerman et al., 1994).

The Knowledge About Breast Cancer Genetics and BRCA1 Testing and the Perceptions of the Benefits, Limitations, and Risks of BRCA1 Testing instruments have been used in research about how high-risk patients will make their decisions about undergoing BRCA1 testing, and the impact of the testing on participants' psychological and functional health status. On the knowledge test, correct answers are added to create a score of 0 to 11 with an average score of 5.97 in one tested population. The percentage of participants responding correctly to individual items ranged from 10% to 75%. Scores for the perception of benefits subscale of the second instrument and the perception of limitations and risks subscale ranged from 6 to 18 with average scores of 15.30 and 8.47, respectively. Further information on scores may be found in Lerman et al. (1996, 1997).

PSYCHOMETRIC PROPERTIES

The instruments were tested with 192 members of families with documented BRCA mutations including both those affected with cancer and those unaffected. The Knowledge Scale showed a Cronbach's alpha of .74.

Factor analysis of the Perceptions of Importance instrument showed two independent factors, "perceptions of benefits (pros)" and "perceptions of limitations/risks (cons)", with Cronbach's alphas of .83 and .81, respectively (Lerman et al., 1996). The finding that baseline knowledge about testing and perceived benefits both related strongly to test use is congruent with what theory would predict and therefore, offers some support for test validity. However, perceived importance of the limitations of risks was not as strongly related as would be expected. Increases in knowledge were significantly greater for women who had closer family relationships with breast or ovarian cancer as compared with women with lesser family involvement. This could be seen as a known groups comparison, supporting validity of the instrument. In a study of 578 women, both instruments were shown to be sensitive to educational and counseling interventions, in comparison with controls (Lerman et al., 1996).

SUMMARY AND CRITIQUE

These instruments are designed to test some of the important elements of informed consent for a condition for which there can be considerable confusion. Although no documentation of content validity could be located, other evidence of validity and reliability is presented.

REFERENCES

Lerman, C., Daly, M., Masny, A., & Balshem, A. (1994). Attitudes about genetic testing for breast-ovarian cancer susceptibility. *Journal of Clinical Oncology, 12,* 843-850.

Lerman, C., Seay, J., Balshem, A., & Audrain, J. (1995). Interest in genetic testing among first-degree relatives of breast cancer patients. *American Journal of Medical Genetics, 57,* 385-392.

Lerman, C., Narod, S., Schulman, K., Hughes, C., Gomez-Caminero, A., Bonney, G., Gold, K., Trock, B., Main, D., Lynch, J., Fulmore, C., Snyder, C., Lemon, S. J., Conway, T., Tonin, P., Lenoir, G., & Lynch, H. (1996). BRCA1 testing in families with hereditary breast-ovarian cancer. *Journal of the American Medical Association, 275,* 1885-1892.

Lerman, C., Biesecker, B., Benkendorf, J. L., Kerner, J., Gomez-Caminero, A., Hughes, C., & Reed, M. M. (1997). Controlled trial of pretest education approaches to enhance informed decision-making for BRCA1 gene testing. *Journal of the National Cancer Institute, 89,* 148-157.

Instrument 3.6

KNOWLEDGE ABOUT BREAST CANCER GENETICS AND BRCA1 TESTING

True items
> Father can pass down an altered BRCA1 gene to his children.
> Woman who does not have an altered BRCA1 gene can still get breast or ovarian cancer.
> Woman who has an altered BRCA1 gene has a higher ovarian cancer risk.
> Sister of a woman with an altered BRCA1 gene has 50% risk of having altered gene.
> Ovarian cancer screening tests often do not detect cancer until after it spreads.
> Woman who has breast removed can still get breast cancer.

False items
> One half of breast cancer cases occur in women who have an altered BRCA1 gene.
> All women who have an altered BRCA1 gene get cancer.
> One in 10 women have an altered BRCA1 gene.
> Having ovaries removed will definitely prevent ovarian cancer.
> Early-onset breast cancer is less likely due to an altered BRCA1 gene than is late-onset breast cancer.

PERCEPTIONS OF THE BENEFITS, LIMITATIONS AND RISKS OF BRCA1 TESTING

	Not at All Important (1)	Some-what Imporant (2)	Very Important (3)
Perceived benefits of BRCA1 testing			
Reassurance			
Enhance cancer prevention			
Learn children's risk			
Make surgery decisions			
Make childbearing decisions			
Increase cancer screening			
Reduce uncertainty			
Perceived limitations and risks of BRCA1 testing			
Insurance discrimination			
Loss of confidentiality			
Stigmatization			
Lack of trust in modern medicine			
Can't prevent cancer			
Negative effect on family			
Couldn't handle it emotionally			

SOURCE: From "Controlled trial of pretest education approaches to enhance informed decision-making for BRCA1 gene testing," by C. Lerman, B. Biesecker, J. L. Benkendorf, J. Kerner, A. Gomez-Caminero, C. Hughes, and M. M. Reed, 1997, *Journal of the National Cancer Institute, 89,* pp. 148-157. Reprinted by permission of Oxford University Press.

DECISION BOARD (DB) COMPREHENSION QUESTIONNAIRE (CQ)

Developed by Laurie M. Elit, Mark N. Levine,
Amiram Gafni, Timothy J. Whelan, Gordon Doig,
David L. Streiner, and Barry Rosen

INSTRUMENT DEVELOPMENT, ADMINISTRATION, AND SCORING

Assuring adequate patient understanding with which to make treatment decisions is important. The Decision Board (DB), seeking to determine preferences, describes two treatment options, their potential side effects, and the possible outcomes to the patient who has completed surgery for suboptimally debulked ovarian cancer. The DB is a standardized method of information transfer and is accompanied by a comprehension questionnaire. Observational study found oncologists giving patients information about their disease status and treatment options, less frequently providing knowledge about side effects, and still less frequently offering facts about survival time. This pattern of response does not provide women with complete information on which to base treatment preferences.

Two oncologists and two clinical epidemiologists were involved in scenario design including definition of domains in which patients require information, with attention to framing of the messages. These domains are present disease status, chemotherapy options, side effects, and survival information. Additional specialists provided further review. Readability level was seventh grade, and the Board was tested for readability and understanding in three women who had completed chemotherapy for ovarian cancer and were disease-free. Review of the DB with patients took 20 to 30 minutes—correct answers to the CQ are summed (Elit et al., 1996). The full DB script and additional details of the study may be found in Elit (1995).

PSYCHOMETRIC PROPERTIES

Psychometric properties were studied in 37 volunteers without cancer, 11 women following first-line chemotherapy for ovarian cancer, and 12 patients with stage IIIc-IV ovarian cancer at the point of deciding future chemotherapy. Anxiety did not change appreciably before and after use of the DB; this finding is an important part of the feasibility of using the instrument. The comprehension questionnaire was answered correctly by nearly all of the healthy volunteers and the patients with ovarian cancer who had completed chemotherapy. After 3 weeks, a different observer interviewed ten of the healthy volunteers (interobserver reliability), with 100% agreement on repeat testing. When probabilities for outcome were systematically changed, most healthy women had predictable shifts in expressed preference, supporting validity of the instrument. The method of presenting survival information (median survival vs. percentage survival at 3.5 years) significantly influenced choice, illustrating the importance of a standard method in research.

At the point of deciding first-line chemotherapy in a poor prognostic situation with ovarian cancer, patients still valued survival more highly than quality of life during chemotherapy.

SUMMARY AND CRITIQUE

The DB, along with the CQ, is used as an intervention tool and as an assessment tool. It may also be used in a take-home version. Content validity should be further studied with patients themselves rather than assuming that physicians know the important areas of women's preferences. Thus far, the DB has been used with small samples and the long-term impact of providing survival information has not been explored. Neither have markers been identified for who should receive this information. Quality-of-life information, which was requested by many of the women studied, was not available to be incorporated; thus, how much quality-of-life information influences choice of treatment could not be studied (Elit et al., 1996). In addition, Elit et al.'s research does not address whether the use of the DB increases comprehensibility compared with standard measures.

The DBs for several other health conditions have been developed and tested for measurement of treatment preferences, including decisions for or against adjuvant chemotherapy for women with node-negative breast cancer deemed to be at high risk for recurrence. The value judgment was whether reduction of the patient's quality of life during treatment was worth a small long-term reduction in risk for recurrence. This DB was developed similarly to that described by Elit et al. (1996) and tested with 30 healthy female volunteers, showing test-retest reliability of .86 and predictable preference shifts when odds were changed. It was then tested with 37 newly presenting patients. Strength of preference was measured on a 6-point Likert scale (Levine, Gafni, Markham, & MacFarlane, 1992).

A DB has also been developed for use by patients with chronic myeloid leukemia who are deciding between the therapeutic alternatives of bone marrow transplant and conservative management during the early phase of disease. Thus far, this DB has been tested with healthy individuals only (Sebban et al., 1995). An additional DB has been developed for patients making a decision about breast irradiation post lumpectomy (Whelan et al., 1995).

REFERENCES

Elit, L. M. (1995). *Design and pretesting of a decision aid to elicit patient preference for treatment of advanced epithelial ovarian cancer.* Unpublished masters thesis, McMaster University, Hamilton, Ontario.

Elit, L. M., Levine, M. N., Gafni, A., Whelan, T. J., Doig, G., Streiner, D. L., & Rosen, B. (1996). Patients' preferences for therapy in advanced epithelial ovarian cancer: Development, testing and application of a bedside decision instrument. *Gynecologic Oncology, 62,* 329-335.

Levine, M. N., Gafni, A., Markham, B., & MacFarlane, D. (1992). A bedside decision instrument to elicit a patient's preference concerning adjuvant chemotherapy for breast cancer. *Annals of Internal Medicine, 117,* 53-58.

Sebban, C., Browman, G., Gafni, A., Norman, G., Levine, M., Assouline, D., & Fiere, D. (1995). Design and validation of a bedside decision instrument to elicit a patient's preference concerning allogenic bone marrow transplantation in chronic myeloid leukemia. *American Journal of Hematology, 48,* 221-227.

Whelan, T. J., Levine, M. N., Gafni, A., Lukka, H., Mohide, E. A., Patel, M., & Streiner, D. L. (1995). Breast irradiation postlumpectomy: Development and evaluation of a decision instrument. *Journal of Clinical Oncology, 13,* 847-853.

Instrument 3.7

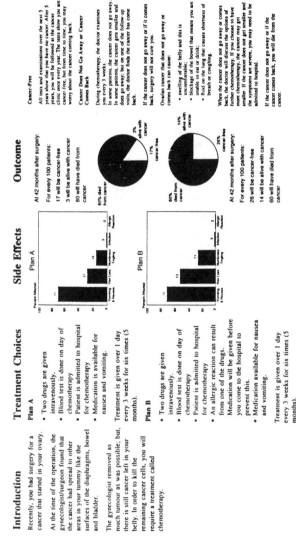

Introduction

Recently, you had surgery for a cancer that started in your ovary.

At the time of the operation, the gynecologist/surgeon found that the cancer had spread to other areas in your tummy like the surfaces of the diaphragms, bowel and bladder.

The gynecologist removed as much tumour as was possible; but, there is still cancer left in your belly. In order to kill the remaining cancer cells, you will require a treatment called chemotherapy.

Treatment Choices

Plan A

- Two drugs are given intravenously.
- Blood test is done on day of chemotherapy
- Patient is admitted to hospital for chemotherapy
- Medication is available for nausea and vomiting.

Treatment is given over 1 day every 3 weeks for six times (5 months).

Plan B

- Two drugs are given intravenously.
- Blood test is done on day of chemotherapy
- Patient is admitted to hospital for chemotherapy
- An allergic reaction can result from one of the drugs. Medication will be given before you come to the hospital to prevent this.
- Medication available for nausea and vomiting.

Treatment is given over 1 day every 3 weeks for six times (5 months).

Side Effects

Plan A

Plan B

Outcome

At 42 months after surgery:

For every 100 patients:
17 will be cancer-free
3 will be alive with cancer
80 will have died from cancer

80% died from cancer
3% alive with cancer
17% cancer-free

At 42 months after surgery:

For every 100 patients:
26 will be cancer-free
14 will be alive with cancer
60 will have died from cancer

60% died from cancer
14% alive with cancer
26% cancer-free

Cancer-Free

All tests and examinations over the next 5 years show that you have no cancer. After 5 years, you will be followed at the cancer clinic once every year. The tests show you are cancer-free, but from time to time, you may worry about the cancer coming back.

Cancer Does Not Go Away or Cancer Comes Back

During chemotherapy, the doctor examines you every 3 weeks.
In some patients, the cancer does not go away.
In some patients, the cancer gets smaller and does go away; but on one of the follow-up visits, the doctor finds the cancer has come back.

If the cancer does not go away or if it comes back, surgery will not cure you.

Ovarian cancer that does not go away or comes back can cause:

- swelling of the belly and this is uncomfortable;
- blockage of the bowel that means you are unable to eat or drink;
- fluid on the lung that causes shortness of breath or coughing.

When the cancer does not go away or comes back, the doctor will discuss the options of further chemotherapy. If you choose to have more chemotherapy, the cancer may get smaller. If the cancer does not get smaller and the symptoms are severe, you may need to be admitted to hospital.

If the cancer does not go away or if the cancer comes back, you will die from the cancer.

SOURCE: From "Patients' preferences for therapy in advanced epithelial ovarian cancer: Development, testing and application of a bedside decision instrument," by L. M. Elit, M. N. Levine, A. Gafni, T. J. Whelan, G. Doig, D. L. Streiner, and B. Rosen, 1996, Gynecologic Oncology, 62, pp. 329-335. Copyright 1996 by Academic Press, Inc. Reprinted by permission.

Instrument 3.8

TABLE 2 Comprehension Questionnaire

The surgeon was able to remove all the cancer in my belly.	True	False
Chemotherapy cures most people with ovarian cancer.	True	False
Chemotherapy will increase the length of my life.	True	False
If the cancer comes back, surgery will cure the cancer.	True	False
Both treatment plans are given for six courses or roughly 5 months.	True	False
One of the plans required that I take medication at home prior to receiving the chemotherapy.	True	False
One plan offers a better cure rate with more side effects.	True	False
The chemotherapy cures a small number of patients. Chemotherapy mainly acts to make the cancer get smaller for a time.	True	False
Chemotherapy will cause some nausea and vomiting.	True	False
Chemotherapy will cause all people to lose all their hair.	True	False

SOURCE: From "Patients' preferences for therapy in advanced epithelial ovarian cancer: Development, testing and application of a bedside decision instrument," by L. M. Elit, M. N. Levine, A. Gafni, T. J. Whelan, G. Doig, D. L. Streiner, and B. Rosen, 1996, *Gynecologic Oncology, 62,* pp. 329-335. Copyright 1996 by Academic Press, Inc. Reprinted by permission.

DEACONESS INFORMED CONSENT COMPREHENSION TEST (DICCT)

Developed by Cheryl K. Miller, Danielle C. O'Donnell,
H. Russell Searight, and Rick A. Barbarash at
Family Medicine Research Center of
Deaconess Hospital, St. Louis, MO

INSTRUMENT DEVELOPMENT, ADMINISTRATION, AND SCORING

Federal regulations mandate that informed consent documents for research contain, at minimum, information regarding eight basic elements: the study's nature and purpose; direct and indirect benefits; discomfort and potential risks; alternative procedures; extent of confidentiality of study records; investigators' willingness to answer participants' questions regarding the study; permission by participants to withdraw without penalty or prejudice; and provision of treatment or compensation for any research-related injury (Miller, O'Donnell, Searight, & Barbarash, 1996).

There is no standard for assessing how much, or even if, a study participant understands the information present. A growing body of data suggests that patient understanding of this information, which is necessary to make an informed choice, is not always achieved. The criteria of recall versus recognition versus retention of information are obviously different and not necessarily synonymous with comprehension. Thus, the DICCT permits subjects to describe the information in their own words rather than requiring a rote recitation of the informed consent document (Miller et al., 1996).

The instrument includes a questionnaire of open-ended items and explicit scoring criteria. Miller et al. believe the questions are written in lay language at the eighth grade reading level. DICCT questions are read verbatim from a script and answers given verbally; therefore, this method is useful for subjects whose literacy and writing skills are poor. Administration requires about 7 minutes and scoring an additional 5 minutes. Responses are scored 2 points = correct answer, 1 point = correct but incomplete answer or one demonstrating poverty of content, and 0 points = incorrect or no answer. Total possible score is 28 points (Miller et al., 1996).

PSYCHOMETRIC PROPERTIES

The DICCT was administered to 275 adults entering one of four ambulatory clinical drug research trials. For 50 subjects, the DICCT was scored by two blinded, trained investigators with an interrater agreement of .84. The questions closely correspond to the informed consent elements, supporting content and face validity. At present, there is no established standard for determining the criterion validity of an instrument such as the DICCT. Correlations of DICCT scores with psychometrically established vocabulary and reading tests and education level were moderate, presumably showing a common core of cognitive skills (Miller et al., 1996).

SUMMARY AND CRITIQUE

Research on informed consent and the conduct of clinical investigators can be enhanced by use of a standardized, psychometrically sound test for assessing participants' understanding of this material. Study investigators are responsible for providing subjects with relevant information but have no duty to ensure they understand it. The DICCT can be used to assess that understanding and then improve it. It can also be used for periodic checks of participant understanding during a long study. Evidence of the DICCT's sensitivity to intervention could not be located.

It is not clear that vocabulary and reading tests and educational level offer good opportunities to test validity. Further evidence of validity would be useful. The DICCT has apparently so far been used only with patients who were young, well educated and not seriously or critically ill, thus likely offering limited generalizability of reliabilty and validity data. A limitation of the DICCT is that some answers are study specific. However, the information that is variable is factual and may be substituted easily (Miller et al., 1996; Searight, Miller, O'Donnell, & Barbarash, n.d.).

The authors of the DICCT rightfully point out that there are no guidelines for how investigators are to proceed if, for purposes of informed consent, a subject's understanding appears deficient. Previous studies show that with increased time retention declines, content about adverse events have the poorest retention rates, and geriatric patients and those with below-average intellectual functioning appear to show more difficulty with comprehension of study material (Searight & Miller, 1996). These concerns highlight important issues at least partially addressed by this instrument.

REFERENCES

Miller, C. K., O'Donnell, D. C., Searight, H. R., & Barbarash, R. A. (1996). The Deaconess Informed Consent Comprehension Test: An assessment tool for clinical research subjects. *Pharmacotherapy, 16*, 872-878.

Searight, H. R., & Miller, C. K. (1996). Remembering and interpreting informed consent: A qualitative study of drug trial participants. *Journal of the American Board of Family Practice, 9*, 14-22.

Searight, H. R., Miller, C. K., O'Donnell, D. C., & Barbarash, R. A. (n. d.). Deaconess Informed Consent Comprehension Test: Summary of psychometric properties and related research.

Instrument 3.9

DEACONESS INFORMED CONSENT
COMPREHENSION TEST

Individual Items

1) What is the purpose of the study?

    2 points—complete answer. Example—to test a new drug used to treat a specific medical condition.

    1 point—to get a new drug approved; to test a new drug; to gather information on a new drug.

    0 points—(any obviously wrong answer); so the investigators/I can make money; so I can get free drugs/treatment.

2) When should you begin using the medication?

    2 points—thorough answer describing all relevant indicators for initiating medication.

    1 point—general answer or incomplete answer.

    0 points—any other answer.

3) After you begin the medication, how often are you supposed to take it?

    2 points—thorough answer.

    1 point—incomplete answer.

    0 points—any other answer.

4) What are the possible risks or discomforts associated with the study?

    2 points—at least *two* specific risks or sources of discomfort.

    1 point—*one* of the above or any side effects that have not yet been reported.

    0 points—any other answer.

5) Describe all benefits that may be expected for you and others as a result of the research.

    2 points—two or more benefits—either general or specific to the subject such as free medication, compensation, or knowledge gained by the study may benefit future patients.

    1 point—any one of the above.

    0 points—any other answer.

6) Besides participating in the study, describe other treatment, if any, available that may be advantageous to you.

   2 points—specific names of other appropriate treatments.

   1 point—recognition that there is another drug or treatment available.

   0 points—nothing; don't know; inappropriate drug for the condition.

7) Who can you contact if you have questions regarding the study and about your rights as a research subject?

   2 points—*two* or more of the following: the investigator/doctor; the study nurse/coordinator; the chairperson of the institutional review board.

   1 point—any *one* of the above.

   0 points—any other answer.

8) If you become physically injured or ill as a direct result of participating in the study, who do you contact?

   2 points—any one of the following: the investigators; the study doctors; the research director; anyone specifically named as a contact for physical illness or injury from study participation.

   1 point—(general answer): the nurse; the research staff; the research office; the doctor.

   0 points—(irrelevant answer): the emergency room; my personal physician.

9) If you become physically injured or ill as a direct result of participating in the study, what compensation is available?

   2 points—any medical treatment/drugs/procedures required will be paid for; my medical bills will be paid/covered.

   1 point—anything I require.

   0 points—there is no compensation if I become ill or injured; none; free medical care only if I continue to participate in the study.

10) If you become physically injured or ill as a direct result of participating in the study, who will pay for any necessary treatment?

   2 points—the drug company or institution sponsoring the research.

   1 point—the study.

   0 points—the investigator/doctor; my insurance; me; nobody.

11) Your participation in the study is voluntary. What will happen if you refuse to be in the study?

   2 points—nothing; it will not be held against me; there is no penalty or consequences; no one would be mad at me.
   1 point—I wouldn't be in the study; I wouldn't get free medicine or medical care or money.
   0 points—I won't come to the office; the doctor/investigators will get mad at me; it would be held against me; I would be penalized; I would have to go to my own doctor; I wouldn't be cured.

12) Your participation in this study is voluntary. What would happen if you agree to participate and later change your mind?

   2 points—I can take myself out/quit/discontinue the study without penalty/ consequences; nothing—I can quit anytime I want to; I will call the in- vestigator/doctors and tell them I don't want to be in the study; I can change my mind and take myself out of the study without penalty.
   1 point—nothing—I will be out of the study.
   0 points—I can't change my mind; once I am in the study I can't get out; investigator/doctors will get mad at me; I call the research office and tell them; I would return the study medication; I wouldn't get paid.

13) How would your decision on whether or not to participate in the study effect your present or future medical care with the study doctors or the institution?

   2 points—my decision on whether or not to be in the study will not affect my present or future medical care by an investigator/doctor/institution; it will not affect my care—I can still be a patient at this institution; the doctors will take care of me/provide me with medical care.
   1 point—the investigators don't care if I participate or not; it won't.
   0 points—I cannot be a patient at this institution if I do not participate in the study; the doctors will not want me as a patient if I do not partici- pate; I would be given "low priority" care.

14) Can you tell me who is allowed to see your medical records for the study?

   2 points—(any *two* of the following): the investigator/doctors; the spon- soring institution; the Food and Drug Administration.
   1 point—any *one* of the above.
   0 points—none of the above.

SOURCE: Developed by Cheryl Miller, Danielle O'Donnell, Rick Barbarash, and H. Russell Searight at the Family Medical Research Center of Deaconess Hospital, St. Louis, MO. Reprinted with permission.

4

Decisional Capacity

Some patients lack the mental capacity to understand or to make choices about their health care. More specifically, they are without the ability to understand and to appreciate the relevance of information for themselves, to rationally manipulate the information, and to express a choice. The term "decisional capacity" is distinguished from the legal term "competency" and refers to the ability to comprehend, evaluate, and choose among realistic options before the patient. Assessment of an individual's capacity should involve only those decisional domains in question. Commonly in health situations, these include the capacity to make treatment decisions, to complete advance directives (ADs), or to participate in research. Detailed guidelines for capacity to complete ADs may be found in Silberfeld, Nash, and Singer (1993). A diagnosis of depression, dementia, delirium, or psychosis does not in itself establish lack of decisional capacity. In many patients, capacity may wax and wane.

Because it is known that clinical impressions can be inaccurate, an instrument with good psychometric characteristics can provide an additional piece of data to be used for judgment about decisional capacity. Stringency of the test and the standard to which the patient is held should vary with the extent and probability of risk and benefit.

To significantly increase their reliability, instruments to assess capacity have been measured against psychiatric assessments according to standard guidelines. An infrequently used alternative in research is to use "normal" control groups as a basis for comparison to those demonstrating impaired capacity. Differentiation between ignorance and lack of decisional capacity requires excellent patient education about the decision topic until understanding can no longer be improved.

Because of fluctuating capacity in many patients, the assessment of decisional capacity should avoid denying patients their autonomy if they are able to make decisions but also to provide for substituted judgment if they cannot. Interventions designed to support decision making in individuals with varying levels of capacity, including those due to health care environments, would be an exciting development.

REFERENCE

Silberfeld, M., Nash, C., & Singer, P. A. (1993). Capacity to complete an advance directive. *Journal of the American Geriatric Society, 41,* 1141-1143.

STANDARDIZED MINI-MENTAL STATE EXAMINATION (SMMSE)

Developed by William Molloy,
Efram Alemayehu,
and Robin Roberts

INSTRUMENT DEVELOPMENT, ADMINISTRATION, AND SCORING

The Mini-Mental Status Exam (MMSE) measures orientation to time and place, immediate recall, short- and long-term memory, calculation, language, constructive ability, and the ability to understand and follow commands. It is the instrument most widely used to measure cognitive impairment in the elderly (Molloy, Alemayehu, & Roberts, 1991). The Standardized Mini-Mental State Examination (SMMSE) standardizes guidelines for administration, scoring, and timing of responses in an effort to increase reliability of the MMSE. Its usefulness in measuring capacity to complete an advance directive (AD) and to consent to treatment is of interest.

Some believe that capacity to complete an advance directive is distinct from capacity to consent to treatment and therefore should be measured differently. To be capable of completing an AD, a person should understand and appreciate that (a) ADs contain choices that will be acted on not in the present but in the future; (b) the choices will be acted on when the person is no longer capable; (c) some of the choices involve medical treatments; (d) some of the choices may involve choosing someone else to make treatment decisions on one's behalf; (e) the choices could result in the person's death or a state of permanent coma, a state in which choice is no longer possible; (f) the person's choices may change over time or as the person's state of health changes, in which case he or she should also change the directive; and (g) the choices in the directive may supersede subsequent choices after the person has become incapable (Silberfeld, Nash, & Singer, 1993).

Others (Etchells et al., 1997) have used the SMMSE to assess patient ($N = 47$) capacity to consent to treatment, finding that a score of 16 or less significantly increased the probability of incapacity against a criterion of psychiatric assessment. However, this score level did continue to misclassify and the authors conclude that the SMMSE scores were not accurate for assessing competency to consent to treatment.

Scores for the SMMSE range from 0 to 30; in a study of 96 individuals from nursing and retirement homes, the mean score was 21.5 and the standard deviation 8.6. Mean time for administration was 10.5 minutes, and the instrument can be administered by trained non-health care providers (Molloy et al., 1996).

PSYCHOMETRIC PROPERTIES

In a study of 48 elderly residents, Molloy et al. found significantly higher interrater and intrarater (.69 and .92, respectively) reliability for the SMMSE than for the MMSE. Two reference standard evaluations were used to judge validity of the SMMSE with 48 patients from a nursing home and a chronic care hospital unit—an assessment by a specially trained nurse in collaboration with an interdisciplinary team and a geriatrician assessment using a decision aid.

Participants were educated about ADs, which allowed people to nominate proxies and specify treatment wishes for life-threatening illness, resuscitation, and feeding. The education was done to increase the possibility of differentiating between ignorance and incompetence.

Very high agreement was found between the SMMSE and the reference standards. An SMMSE cutoff score of 20 was believed to accurately classify individuals who had been thoroughly educated to be capable or incapable of making AD decisions (although no direct evidence of learning was apparently obtained). Use of the SMMSE improved reliability over the MMSE from .69 to .90. Reliability across time with the same rater and across raters was .92 and .90 versus .69 and .69 for the MMSE.

SUMMARY AND CRITIQUE

Molloy et al. indicate that the SMMSE may be applied as a screening test for clinical trials and as an outcome measure. It also differentiates accurately between people who can learn and ultimately complete ADs from those who cannot (Molloy & Standish, 1997).

Findings thus far show the SMMSE to be more reliable than is the MMSE. The SMMSE must also be tested with institutionalized older people, those living in the community, and the mentally ill; reliability may vary in these populations from the chronic care nursing home group with which the instrument has been studied. The findings reported above reflect an assessment of its usefulness for determining capacity to complete an AD that included instructional and proxy components. The capacity required to nominate a proxy is likely to be considerably less than that required to complete a detailed directive. In addition, the usefulness of the SMMSE and the cut score for other relevant decision capacities would need to be established (Molloy et al., 1996).

Clinical tests of capacity can take the form of guidelines for a clinical interview, the use of psychometric tests, and direct evaluation of decisional abilities (such as the permissible error approach). The appropriate threshold is always a question. Some have agreed that the capacity to develop an AD should have the same threshold as capacity to write a will. How people are selected for testing is also important. The loss of rights should not be a consequence of mere selection for the testing of mental capacity (Silberfeld & Corber, 1996). Assessment of capacity with the SMMSE does not negate the responsibility to educate the patient about ADs and their particular situations.

REFERENCES

Etchells, E., Katz, M. R., Shuchman, M., Wong, G., Workman, S., Choudhry, N. K., Craven, J., & Singer, P. A. (1997). Accuracy of clinical impressions and Mini-Mental State Exam scores for assessing capacity to consent to major medical treatment. *Psychosomatics, 38,* 239-245.

Molloy, D. W., Alemayehu, E., & Roberts, R. (1991). Reliability of a standardized mini-mental state examination compared with the traditional mini-mental state examination. *American Journal of Psychiatry, 148,* 102-105.

Molloy, D. W., Silberfeld, M., Darzins, P., Guyatt, G. H., Singer, P. A., Rush, B., Bedard, M., & Strang, D. (1996). Measuring capacity to complete an advance directive. *Journal of the American Geriatrics Society, 44,* 660-664.

Molloy, D. W., & Standish, T. I. M. (1997). Mental status and neuropsychological assessment: A guide to the Standardized Mini-Mental State Examination. *International Psychogeriatrics, 9*(Suppl. 1), 87-94.

Silberfeld, M., & Corber, W. (1996). Permissible errors in managing property: An approach to the threshold of capacity. *Canadian Journal of Psychiatry, 41,* 513-518.

Silberfeld, M., Nash, C., & Singer, P. A. (1993). Capacity to complete an advance directive. *Journal of the American Geriatrics Society, 41,* 1141-1143.

Instrument 4.1

STANDARDIZED MINI-MENTAL
STATE EXAMINATION (SMMSE)

Dr. D. W. Molloy and Staff
GERIATRIC RESEARCH GROUP
McMaster University

See Reference:

Molloy DW, Alemayehu E, Roberts R. A Standardized Mini-Mental State Examination (SMMSE): Its reliability compared to the traditional Mini-Mental State Examination (MMSE). The American Journal of Psychiatry, Vol. 148:102-105, 1991.

Acknowledgment:

We would like to thank Dr. Marshall Folstein for allowing us to standardize his instrument. His support is greatly appreciated.

Directions for Administration of SMMSE

1.   Before the Questionnaire is administered, try to get the subject to sit down facing you. Assess the subject's ability to hear and understand very simple conversation, e.g., *What is your name?* If the subject uses hearing or visual aids, provide these before starting.

2.   Introduce yourself and try to get the subject's confidence. Before you commence, get the subject's permission to ask questions, e.g., *Would it be all right to ask you some questions about your memory?* This helps to avoid catastrophic reactions.

3.   Ask each question a maximum of three times. If the subject does not respond—score 0.

4.   If the subject answers incorrectly—score 0. Do not hint, prompt or ask the question again, e.g., *What year is this?*—1952. Accept that answer—do not ask the question again, hint or provide any physical clues such as head shaking, etc.

5.   The following equipment is required to administer the instrument: a watch, a pencil, and some blank paper. A piece of paper with CLOSE YOUR EYES is written in large letters and two 5-sided figures intersecting to make a 4-sided figure is also required. We have laminated this paper and enclosed it for your convenience.

6.   If the subject answers *What did you say?*—do not explain or engage in conversation—merely repeat the same directions (e.g. *What year is this?*) to a maximum of 3 times.

7.   If the subject interrupts e.g., *What is this for?*—just reply: *I will explain in a few minutes when we are finished. Now if we could just proceed please. . . . we are almost finished.*

Standardized Mini-Mental State Examination (SMMSE)

I am going to ask you some questions and give you some problems to solve.
Please try to answer as best as you can.

	Max Score

1. **(Allow 10 seconds for each reply)**
   a) *What year is this?* (accept exact answer only) **1**
   b) *What season is this?* (during last week of the old season or first week of a new season, accept either season) **1**
   c) *What month of the year is this?* (on the first day of new month, or last day of the previous month, accept either) **1**
   d) *What is today's date?* (accept previous or next date, e.g., on the 7th accept the 6th or 8th) **1**
   e) *What day of the week is this?* (accept exact answer only) **1**

2. **(Allow 10 seconds for each reply)**
   a) *What county are we in?* (accept exact answer only) **1**
   b) *What province/state/country are we in?* (accept exact answer only) **1**
   c) *What city/town are we in?* (accept exact answer only) **1**
   d) **(In clinic)** *What is the name of this hospital/building?* (accept exact name of hospital or institution only) **1**
      (In home) What is the street address of this house? (accept street name and house number or equivalent in rural areas) **1**
   e) **(In clinic)** *What floor of the building are we on?* (accept exact answer only) **1**
      (In home) What room are we in? (accept exact answer only) **1**

3. **I am going to name 3 objects. After I have said all three objects, I want you to repeat them. Remember what they are because I am going to ask you to name them again in a few minutes.**

   (say them slowly at approximately 1 second intervals) **3**

   Ball   Car   Man

   For repeated use:

Bell	**Jar**	**Fan**
Bill	**Tar**	**Can**
Bull	**War**	**Pan**

Please repeat the 3 items for me.
(score 1 point for each correct reply on the first attempt)

Allow 20 seconds for reply, if subject did not repeat all 3, repeat until they are learned or up to a maximum of 5 times.

**Max
Score**

4. *Spell the word WORLD.*
(you may help subject to spell world correctly)   **5**

Say *now spell it backwards please.* Allow 30 seconds to spell backwards. (If the subject cannot spell world even with assistance—score 0.)

5. *Now what were the 3 objects that I asked you to remember?*   **3**

Ball   Car   Man

Score 1 point for each correct response regardless of order, allow 10 seconds.

6. Show wristwatch. Ask: *what is this called?*   **1**

Score 1 point for correct response. Accept "wristwatch" or "watch". Do not accept "clock", "time", etc. (allow 10 seconds).

7. Show pencil. Ask: *what is this called?*   **1**

Score 1 point for correct response, accept pencil only—score 0 for pen.

8. *I'd like you to repeat a phrase after me: "no if's, and's or but's".*   **1**

(allow 10 seconds for response. Score 1 point for a correct repetition. Must be **exact**, e.g. no if's or but's—score 0)

9. *Read the words on this page and then do what it says:*   **1**

Hand subject the laminated sheet with CLOSE YOUR EYES on it.

CLOSE YOUR EYES

If subject just reads and does not then close eyes—you may repeat: *read the words on this page and then do what it says* to a maximum of 3 times. Allow 10 seconds, score 1 point **only** if subject closes eyes. Subject does not have to read aloud.

	Max Score

10. Ask if the subject is right or left handed. **3**

Alternate right/left hand in statement, e.g., if the subject is right-handed say *Take this paper in your left hand . . .* Take a piece of paper—hold it up in front of subject and say the following:

"Take this paper in your right/left hand, fold the paper in half once with both hands and put the paper down on the floor."

Takes paper in correct hand **1**
Folds it in half **1**
Puts it on the floor **1**

Allow 30 seconds. Score 1 point for each instruction correctly executed.

11. Hand subject a pencil and paper. **1**

Write any complete sentence on that piece of paper.

Allow 30 seconds. Score 1 point. The sentence should make sense. Ignore spelling errors.

12. Place design, pencil, eraser and paper in front of the subject. **1**

Say: *copy this design please.*

Allow multiple tries until patient is finished and hands it back. Score 1 point for correctly copied diagram. The subject must have drawn a 4-sided figure between two 5-sided figures. Maximum time—1 minute.

Total Test Score 30

SCORING THE FIGURE

The subject must draw two 5-sided figures intersected by a 4-sided figure.

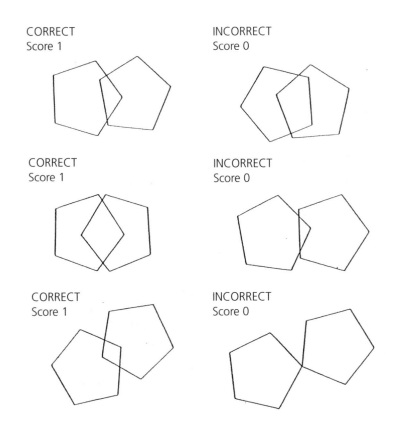

CORRECT
Score 1

INCORRECT
Score 0

CORRECT
Score 1

INCORRECT
Score 0

CORRECT
Score 1

INCORRECT
Score 0

Time completed: _____(minutes)

SCORING "WORLD" BACKWARDS

Correct response: DLROW   **Score 5**

Omission of one letter
  e.g. DLRW; DLOW; DROW; DLRO   **Score 4**

Omission of two letters:
e.g. DLR; LRO; DLW   **Score 3**

Reversal of two letters:
e.g. DLORW; DRLOW; DLRWO; DLWOR   **Score 3**

Omission/reversal of three letters:
e.g. DORLW; DL, OW   **Score 2**

Reversal of four letters:
e.g. DRLWO; LDRWO   **Score 1**

'Serial Sevens'

Alternately the calculation task 'Serial Sevens' may be used instead of WORLD. Decide at the start to use Serial Sevens or WORLD. Do not use Serial Sevens if subject unable to spell WORLD and vice versa.

Say: *"Subtract 7 from 100 and keep subtracting seven from what's left until I tell you to stop"*

(may repeat three times if subject pauses—   **5**
just repeat the same instruction—allow one minute)

Scoring of Serial Sevens: (write down subject's reply)

Once subject starts—do not interrupt—allow him/her to proceed until five subtractions have been made. If subject stops before five subtractions have been made repeat the original instruction "keep subtracting seven from what's left". (maximum 3 times)

Score as follows:

93, 86, 79, 72, 65	5 points (all correct)
93, 88, 81, 74, 67	4 points (4 correct, 1 wrong)
92, 85, 78, 71, 64	4 points (4 correct, 1 wrong)
93, 87, 80, 73, 64	3 points (3 correct, 2 wrong)
92, 85, 78, 71, 63	3 points (3 correct, 2 wrong)
93, 87, 80, 75, 67	2 points (2 correct, 3 wrong)
93, 87, 81, 75, 69	1 point (1 correct, 4 wrong)

Total SMMSE Scores:

24 – 30	Normal range	
20 – 23	Mild	
10 – 19	Moderate	Cognitive impairment
0 – 9	Severe	

INTERPRETING THE SMMSE

These are general guidelines to interpret the SMMSE scores. There is great individual variability.

General

- Serial SMMSE scores provide the best information about a person's function. If in doubt about the significance of a mild memory problem, score the SMMSE every six months.

- Score of 30 indicates no impairment. People with higher education with no obvious sensory, language or communication problems usually score 30.

- Scores of 24 or more are within the range of "normal" in the general population.

- Patients who score in the range of 20-23 have cognitive impairment but can usually still live independently.

- Patients who score less than 20 usually cannot live independently. They tend to have problems with Instrumental Activities of Daily Living such as managing finances, driving, shopping, meal preparation and medications. They usually can manage basic activities of daily living such as grooming, dressing, and eating.

- Some patients' scores may be higher or lower than the norm for actual level of impairment, e.g. patients with higher education tend to score higher; patients with speech or language impairment tend to score lower. This apparent discrepancy between score and functional level is referred to as the "disability gap."

Alzheimer's Disease

- Usually the first deficit is in short-term memory—cannot recall the three items (task #5) after interruption.

- Disorientation to time is followed by disorientation to place. Language deficits start to appear late.

Stroke

- Deficits are more patchy. May have speech/language problems earlier than in Alzheimer's.

Depression

These patients often seem less distressed than Alzheimer's patients about their problems. Alzheimer's patients usually continue to try to get the right answer. Patients with depression are more likely to answer: "I don't know" or "It doesn't matter". When pressed they often know the answer but couldn't be bothered.

They may have somatic complaints in the bowels. They may also have a "disability gap", performing much worse than you think they should. In conversation they do not have the obvious short-term memory loss or word finding difficulties of the Alzheimer patient, but score low on the test. Suspect depression if the patient also displays any of the following symptoms: change of appetite, energy loss, sleep disturbance, weight loss, loss of libido and mention of suicide.

Developing the Care Plan:

Knowledge of the level of cognitive loss guides a care plan. Individualize the care plan so the person will not fail at functions/performance that are too complex, yet allows the patient to function at his/her maximum potential.

Problems with judgment: get a power of attorney, advance directive and start building a support network.

Short term memory loss: use reminders, lists, cues, calendars, diaries.

Language difficulties: avoid open ended questions: instead of "What would you like to drink?", use "Would you like juice or water?" Avoid idiomatic expressions e.g. "Get off my case."

Word finding problems: try to keep language simple, give adequate time to respond, communicate one idea at a time and avoid words with more than one meaning e.g. ceiling/sealing.

3-Step command deficit: give one instruction and one idea at a time. Instead of "Let's go for a walk." try, "Can you stand up please? Now come this way. Let's put your coat on. Now let's go outside."

Repeats "no if, and or but": consider high frequency hearing loss.

SMMSE Scores, Stages of Disease and
Areas of Impairment in Alzheimer's Disease

Stages of Cognitive Impairment

Score	May be normal 30-24	Mild 23-20	Moderate 19-10	Severe 9-0
Stage	May be normal	Early	Middle	Late
Duration of stage		0 ⇒ 2-3 years	⇒ 4-7 years	⇒ 7-14 years

Area of Impairment

Score	May be normal 30-24	Mild 23-20	Moderate 19-10	Severe 9-0
Activities of daily living		Driving, finances, shopping	Dressing, grooming, toileting	Eating, walking
Communication		Word-finding, repeating, goes off topic	Sentence fragments, vague terms (e.g. This, that)	Speech disturbances (e.g. Stuttering, slurring)
Memory		Three item recall, orientation (time, then place)	World spelling, language and 3-step command	All areas show obvious deficits

SMMSE Answer Sheet

Section 1

1.	Year	❏ 1	6.	Country	❏ 1
2.	Season	❏ 1	7.	Province/state/city	❏ 1
3.	Month	❏ 1	8.	City/town	❏ 1
4.	Today's date	❏ 1	9.	Place	❏ 1
5.	Day of the week	❏ 1	10.	Floor of the building	❏ 1

Section 2

11.	Word 1	❏ 1	16.	No if's, and's or but's	❏ 1
	Word 2	❏ 1	17.	Subject closes eyes	❏ 1
	Word 3	❏ 1	18.	Takes paper in correct hand	❏ 1
12.	DLROW or	❏ 5		Folds it in half	❏ 1
	Serial Sevens			Puts it on the floor	❏ 1
13.	Word 1	❏ 1	19.	Sentence	❏ 1
	Word 2	❏ 1	20.	Four-sided figure in two five-sided figures	❏ 1
14.	Wristwatch	❏ 1			
15.	Pencil	❏ 1		**Total score**	❏ 30

SMMSE ANSWER SHEET

Patient's name _____   Date _____

Section 1

1.	Year	[ ] 1	6.	Country	[ ] 1
2.	Season	[ ] 1	7.	Province/State/County	[ ] 1
3.	Month	[ ] 1	8.	City/Town	[ ] 1
4.	Today's date	[ ] 1	9.	Place	[ ] 1
5.	Day of the week	[ ] 1	10.	Floor of Building	[ ] 1

Section 2

11.	Word 1	[ ] 1	16.	No if's, and's or but's	[ ] 1
	Word 2	[ ] 1	17.	Subject closes eyes	[ ] 1
	Word 3	[ ] 1	18.	Takes paper in correct hand	[ ] 1
12.	DLROW or	[ ] 5		Folds it in half	[ ] 1
	Serial Sevens			Puts it on the floor	[ ] 1
13.	Word 1	[ ] 1	19.	Sentence	[ ] 1
	Word 2	[ ] 1	20.	4-sided figure in 2 five-sided figures	[ ] 1
	Word 3	[ ] 1			
14.	Wristwatch	[ ] 1			
15.	Pencil	[ ] 1		Total Score	[ ] 30

Close
Your
Eyes

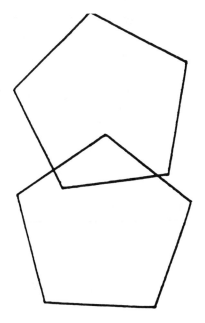

5 Advance Directives

Advance directives (ADs) are an important way to project patient preferences to a time when they may be incapable of expressing their preferences. Living wills are specific directives about medical procedures that should be either provided for or foregone in specific circumstances. A durable power of attorney for health care is a legal document in which one person assigns another the authority to perform specified actions on behalf of the signer. The power is "durable" because unlike the usual power of attorney, it continues in effect if the signer of the document becomes incompetent (Beauchamp & Childress, 1994).

The authority for various kinds of ADs varies by jurisdiction. In 1990, Congress passed legislation (the Patient Self-Determination Act or PSDA) requiring that all health care institutions receiving federal funds ask patients at the time of admission whether they have ADs and that these patients are given information about them.

Although legally sufficient, difficulties with ADs from an ethical perspective have centered on a lack of sufficient detail to provide guidance about patient preference in particular situations. The instruments in this section use different approaches to further specify ADs and to study how they might be improved. As clinical assessment and research instruments, they should be psychometrically strong. Some use stories or a history approach to further describe patient values. To be specific about decisions that will be faced, others limit the AD to a particular disease. Many are seen as ethically justified clinical instruments intended to be used as an adjunct to legal ADs. These include discussions with families and by surrogates who have too little information about the preferences of the person for whom they are now entrusted to make important decisions. Yet, such approaches also have their weaknesses; for example, elicited values or responses to particular scenarios may be too general to direct an inference of patient choice in a particular situation.

Clearly, research with these or other instruments is essential. Such work should incorporate longitudinal studies to trace changes in values and preferences as patients face new situations. Understanding the impact of various interventions that encourage the use of ADs and the prevention of ethical conflict should also be addressed. Furthermore, these instruments can be used to describe treatment preferences of populations of patients, thus helping to inform institutional and public policy.

REFERENCE

Beauchamp, T. L., & Childress, J. F. (1994). *Principles of biomedical ethics* (4th ed.). New York: Oxford University Press.

VALUES ASSESSMENT AND DIRECTIVES FORM (VAD)

Developed by Rita Kielstein and Hans-Martin Sass

INSTRUMENT DEVELOPMENT, ADMINISTRATION, AND SCORING

Kielstein and Sass (1993) describe three phases in the evolution of advance directives—the legal phase, the checklist phase, and the story phase. The legal phase focuses on the technicalities of constitutional and penal law regarding privacy and professional conduct and has resulted in court decisions and the Patient Self-Determination Act (PSDA). During the checklist phase, instruments are primarily lists asking patients to select from, to assign priorities (or both) to value statements, treatment preferences, and quality-of-life questions (Kielstein & Sass, 1993).

The Values Assessment and Directives Form (VAD) is an example of the story approach. This story-based value assessment is intended for use with healthy, competent individuals. It is designed to encourage a narrative response: (a) rewriting the stories so that the outcome reflects as many of the reader's wishes, values, and preferences as possible and (b) eliciting preferences for current and future treatment (Kielstein & Sass, 1993).

The VAD and checklist-type instruments were tested with 80 respondents (15 patients in dialysis, 15 members of their families, 15 clinicians, and 35 students of medicine and philosophy). Kielstein and Sass indicate that the vast majority of respondents were very reluctant to rewrite the stories although they would tell them in dialogue with a counselor. It is expected that patients' responses to the stories will be integrated into the ongoing dialogue with their physicians. The physician's evaluation summary offers an opportunity to integrate the information from both the stories and the values assessment exercise. Furthermore, it provides a determination of the consistency and clarity of the patient's value profile and the preferences and directives given for future treatment (Kielstein & Sass, 1993).

No analysis or scoring guidelines could be located, although clearly scores could be developed from the numerical responses to the assessment section as well as to the clusters of questions in the physician's evaluation summary.

PSYCHOMETRIC PROPERTIES

The five scenarios were selected because they were believed to be indicative of the variety of cases in which advance directives (ADs) are particularly important (dementia, terminal illness, multimorbidity, progressive chronic illness, and sudden trauma or severe injury). The three questions following each story are believed to represent the 15 most important issues in proxy decision making and ADs. Kielstein and Sass believe that having the competent patient develop the stories rather than extracting value statements by paternalistically leading a discussion is the most valid method for making the patient be the primary moral agent in his or her self- assessment and self-determination.

SUMMARY AND CRITIQUE

Kielstein and Sass note that other story-based and narrative forms would have to be developed for other groups of patients such as those in early stages of chronic disease or terminal illness and those of borderline competence. No formal assessment of content or other validity for both the scenarios and the questions could be located.

Assessment instruments based on lists are obviously easier to score, leading to numbers that can be manipulated statistically. But story completion methods could also yield scores that could in turn help test the hypotheses that the stories more closely resemble the patient's values and preferences as well as respondent comfort (i.e., this method better reflects their values). As presently developed, the VAD appears intended for use with individual patients to elicit values with minimal quantification of their content and to apply those values to their ADs. Yet, even simple categories for analysis of patient response to questions at the end of each scenario of stories rewritten by patients could be used to describe common themes across patients.

In the same manner, categories of description across scenarios could be developed and studied for their predictive value at the time actual decisions had to be made. Having patients rewrite the scenarios provides more individualized responses than do common set responses, which should enhance the accuracy of the prediction.

As currently developed, the rough scoring system could allow comparison of patients' current values and those they would want to have govern future decisions. Study of whatever discrepancies occur between these categories over time and the occurrence of particular events would be very helpful. Indeed, respondents in Kielstein and Sass's study (1993) did show current differences. Nearly 90% said that being without pain was important but as a guide for future proxy decisions, one respondent said it would depend on the situation. Similarly, living as long as possible was important, but two thirds reported that it would depend on the situation.

REFERENCE

Kielstein, R., & Sass, H.-M. (1993). Using stories to assess values and establish medical directives. *Kennedy Institute of Ethics Journal, 3*, 303-325.

Instrument 5.1

I. VALUE ASSESSMENT AND DIRECTIVES
FORM TO BE GIVEN TO THE PATIENT

Stories for Self-Evaluation and Self-Determination

Introduction

Here are five stories of patients at the end of their lives. These stories of disease, suffering, and dying are as different as the patients' life stories are. Most of us have difficulty thinking about the final stages of our own life stories for understandable reasons. But medical history is part of personal history. The stories of our last days will one day become a part of the stories of our own lives. Our own future stories may be full of rich and enjoyable events, but there will also be dark hours of weakness, unexpected harm, pain, and reduced physical and mental mobility.

Early on we should reflect on those personal values, wishes, and preferences that we expect to have guide our medical treatment decisions. Value assessments and advance directives executed prior to acute situations strengthen our capacity for self-evaluation and self-determination in situations of dementia, coma, severe pain, agony, and dying. It is better to develop and clearly express our own ideas, values, and preferences for those dark hours, so that others—family and friends, physicians and nurses—will have advice, guidance, or direction for our future life story.

You may use these stories in different ways. (1) Evaluate the stories in a quiet moment or discuss them with family and friends; this will help you to reflect on those values and wishes that you want to have govern your treatment in comparable situations. (2) You might want to rewrite the stories the way you would like your own future story to read. Feel challenged to put your story, comments, preferences, and directives in writing. (3) Finally, if you want, you may name and direct others to care for you based on your preferences and directives as they are told and expressed here, should situations arise in which you become unable to decide for yourself.

While these five stories challenge you to recollect and to reaffirm those values that are essential for you, an introductory part asks you to reflect on your own experiences with disease, dying, and the hospital setting. A final section allows for value statements and directives. You might want to discuss these stories and your comments with family and friends, as well as with your physician. From time to time, after new insights and experiences, you may want to review the stories and change your comments or directives.

Recollection

Stories of fatal disease, suffering, and dying are catalysts for the recollection of one's own, often unpleasant and agonizing, experiences. Many of us have our own stories to tell, stories that have already become a part of our own life histories. What are your stories? What has become a part of your life story?

1. Have I been in the hospital? Why? How long?
2. Has my own suffering or the accidents or diseases of loved ones or friends become a part of my own history and influenced my understanding of disease and pain? What has influenced me?
3. Have I been a witness to death and dying? What were my reactions and impressions? What still moves me?

Five Stories for Self-Evaluation and Self-Determination

Story 1: Who Shall Die? How Should It Be Decided?

Mr. B. is 79-years-old and dependent on others. His eyesight and hearing have diminished. He seems to have lost all interest in life. At times he is very confused and does not even recognize others. He has pain in his legs and can only walk short distances because of poor blood supply to his legs, which is caused by previous smoking. Blood vessel surgery might improve his mobility and reduce the pain, thus improving his quality of life. Mr. B. does not understand the situation nor can he make his preferences clear; he does not have an "advance directive." Two of his sons and the physician favor surgery while his third son is opposed.

1. If you were in Mr. B.'s situation, unable to decide for yourself, who should decide for you, your son or daughter, both together, your spouse or friend, your physician, who else? Give names and addresses.
2. Should physicians follow advance directives? Do you have one? Do you want your comments on this form to serve as an advance directive?
3. How would you have wished to be treated?
4. Rewrite the story the way you would like it to end!

Story 2: Dying of Incurable Cancer?

Mrs. M., 38-years-old, had her left breast removed five years ago because she had breast cancer. Now she has increasing pain in her lower back, and her physicians have determined that the cancer has metastasized to her bones. They recommend chemotherapeutic treatment to reduce pain and to prevent or to slow down further spread of the cancer. Mrs. M. undergoes chemotherapy with uncomfortable side effects. Her pain increases and is not treated adequately. The physicians do not tell her the "full truth," that chemotherapy will not cure her cancer, but might prolong her life. Mrs. M. dies in the hospital eight months after the cancer in her bones was detected; she did not die at home as she had wished. Without chemotherapy she might have died a few months earlier.

1. How would you have wished to be treated?
2. Would you want your physicians to fully inform you about your condition, even if it is fatal?
3. Would you want intensive and aggressive pain treatment, even if it might reduce your mental alertness?
4. Rewrite the story the way you would like it to end!

Story 3: Selecting the Cause of Your Death?

Mr. D., 44-years-old and a diabetic for more than 30 years, has to inject himself with insulin daily and has to obey a strict diet. Four years ago he became blind, a late result of diabetes. Two years ago he became a patient in his neighborhood dialysis center and had to be connected to the "artificial kidney" machine for a couple of hours three times a week. When he became a dialysis patient, he first refused treatment and expressed his wish to die. A year ago, his left leg had to be taken off. He consented to surgery because it was lifesaving and because he wanted to live long enough to be present at his daughter's wedding and to see his first grandchild. Now, lifesaving amputation of his left arm is mandated. This time he refuses surgery and the continuation of dialysis treatment against the strong and repeated recommendations of his physicians. He slowly glides into a coma and dies, as he had wished, ten days after his last dialysis treatment.

1. How would you have decided?
2. What arguments support your decision?
3. Under what circumstances would you want to prolong life by continuing intensive treatment?
4. Rewrite the story the way you would like it to end!

Story 4: Losing the Will to Live

Mrs. S., 80-years-old, is alert and competent but suffers from heart pain and arthritis, in addition to her often painful and incurable intestine inflammation. Her two sons are living in another state. Since her husband died two years ago, she has lost the will to live. She told her family physician about her plans to commit suicide and asked that her decision be respected. Now, she calls the doctor and tells him that she has taken the necessary pills and wants to die in peace and not be revived or put into the hospital. A few hours later, the doctor makes a house call. No one opens the door, and a neighbor lets him into Mrs. S.'s apartment. They find her lying on the couch unconscious and a note on the table reading, "Please, let me die!" The doctor follows her wishes. A court did not hold him responsible for not saving her life.

1. Can you imagine that you would act like Mrs. S. in similar situations?
2. Would you want your doctor to give you detailed information on how to commit suicide or even assist you in doing so?

3. How do you evaluate the doctor's reaction in moral and in legal terms?
4. Rewrite the story the way you would like it to end!

Story 5: Questionable Intervention Following a Severe Accident

Mr. T., 45-years-old, was burned in a severe car accident. More than 50 percent of his skin is burned. He is being treated unsuccessfully in specialized intensive care. Because of effective pain treatment, Mr. T. is mostly sedated and does not recognize his environment. He dies ten months after the accident. If he had survived, he would not have been able to see, as both eyes were burned severely, nor would he have been able to use his severely burned hands. When the physicians initiated treatment, they were aware of those lasting effects.

1. How would you wish to be treated in this or similar situations?
2. What arguments do you have for your decision?
3. What are the mental or physical handicaps that might cause you to wish to be dead rather than alive?
4. Rewrite the story the way you would like it to end!

Which Values and Wishes Shall Govern Your Treatment?

These five stories show conflicts between the capabilities of medical technology and individual preferences and wishes. Others might not make the correct proxy decisions when deciding for you. Therefore you should let them know about your preferences and give them directions. Tell them which values and wishes you would prefer to have govern the last days and hours of your life story.

Indicate, using the scale of one to five, the importance of each of the following eight general value statements as an indicator of your current values and, using the scale of A to E, indicate whether you want the same eight statements to be used by a proxy to govern future treatment decisions were you to become incompetent. [Note: Selecting "A" would mean that it is "very important" for your proxy to use your current value preference in making future decisions for you, whereas selecting "E" would mean that your proxy should not consider your current value preference in making future decisions. For example, if you definitely would *not* want "to live as long as possible" were you permanently unconscious and if it is very important that your proxy use that value preference in making decisions for you, then you would select "5" and "A" for the first value statement.]

Current Value Assessment
1—Yes, very important
2—Important
3—Not important
4—I cannot decide
5—No

Future Decision Making
A—Yes, very important
B—Important
C—Depending on situation
D—I cannot decide
E—No

1. I want to live as long as possible	1,2,3,4,5	A,B,C,D,E
-if I am permanently unconscious	1,2,3,4,5	A,B,C,D,E
-if I am mentally incompetent	1,2,3,4,5	A,B,C,D,E
-if I am terminally ill	1,2,3,4,5	A,B,C,D,E
2. I want to be without pain	1,2,3,4,5	A,B,C,D,E
3. I do not want to be dependent	1,2,3,4,5	A,B,C,D,E
4. I do not want to die in the hospital	1,2,3,4,5	A,B,C,D,E
5. I want a comfortable dying process	1,2,3,4,5	A,B,C,D,E
6. I do not want to be left alone	1,2,3,4,5	A,B,C,D,E
7. I do not want to be a burden	1,2,3,4,5	A,B,C,D,E
8. I want my values to govern treatment	1,2,3,4,5	A,B,C,D,E

If you intend this to be a legally binding advance directive, please sign it and have it witnessed according to the laws of your state. If you change your story, comments, or directives, do so in writing by dating and signing those changes. It is always a good idea to review stories, comments, and directives from time to time and to sign and date them again, even if you do not change anything, as this would indicate your repeated commitment to previous statements.

If you wish, please include comments on these and other stories, wishes, or preferences on additional pages.

Additional Comments, Wishes, Directives:

SIGNED

WITNESSED   DATED

II. EVALUATION SUMMARY FOR THE PHYSICIAN

The story-based Value Assessment and Directives Form (VAD) does not provide ready made prescriptions for providing, withdrawing, or withholding life-sustaining treatment. Rather, the VAD supplies additional essential information on a patient's value profile and life perspective, which, in combination with medical status results, should be used to design patient-oriented treatment. Only integrated information from a value history and medical history permits medically and ethically sound treatment and proxy decision making. The VAD is best established in non-acute situations, and annual physical checkups routinely should include a review of the VAD.

The Value Assessment and Directives Form has three sections. The first section allows the patient to recollect previous experiences and values associated with suffering and dying and to express his/her emotions and feelings. It provides information on the depth of experience on which the patient's comments and directives are based. The second, and central, section confronts the patient with five scenarios—called stories—including dementia, incurable cancer, endstage chronic disease, suicide, and marginally beneficial intervention, and calls for a spontaneous and direct response in expressing values, wishes, preferences, and directives. The third section addresses eight value questions under two different perspectives, current values and advance directives, thus giving the patient input into the widely debated question of how far actual value preferences should govern future interventions.

Physician's Evaluation Summary

This evaluation summary refers to S (the stories) and V (the value statements) in the patient's Value Assessment and Directives Form. Equal attention should be given to patients' rewriting of the stories, comments, and value preference indications.

1. Does the patient have an advance directive? [S1.2; V8]
2. Is this value assessment her/his advance directive? [S1.2; V]
3. Has the patient chosen a proxy decision maker? [S1.1; V8]
4. How closely shall the patient's directives be followed? [S1; V 1-8]
5. How does the patient evaluate life-sustaining treatment in terminal care? [S2; S3; V1]
6. How does the patient evaluate medical intervention of marginal or questionable benefit? [S1; S2; S5]
7. How does the patient feel about "truth-telling," particularly in terminal cases? [S2.2]
8. How does the patient value palliative care, even if it would shorten life or reduce mental capability? [S2; S5; V2]
9. How does the patient classify suicide? [S4; (S3); V8]
10. How does the patient judge physician-assisted or -tolerated suicide? [S4]
11. What are the patient's preferences and directives for medical assistance in the process of dying? [S2; S3; S4; V2; V4; V5; V6]
12. How important are family, social integration, and/or home environment to the patient? [S2; S3; S4; V3; V4; V6]
13. Does the patient consider financial or other burdens on his or her family or friends? [V7]
14. *General Evaluation I:* How consistent is the patient's value profile?
15. *General Evaluation II:* How far can this value profile be used as the patient's advance directive?

Test Scenarios

The following "test scenarios" can be used to test, support, and strengthen the information in the VAD.

Test Story A:

You are brought to the hospital with internal bleeding following a car accident. Immediate surgery stops the bleeding of the liver. However, during surgery tissue suspected to be cancerous is found in the peritoneal cavity. Instant diagnosis confirms the presence of incurable cancer. The immediate removal of visible cancerous tissue and subsequent aggressive treatment might prolong your life by a few months but will reduce your quality of life. What should be done? Who should decide?

[Testing: S1.1-3; S2.1; S3.3; S5; V1-4, 7-8; PES 1-6, 12-15]

Expected response:

Actual response:

Physician's comment:

Test Story B:

You are 62-years-old and suffer from progressive symptoms of Alzheimer's disease. You do not recognize where you are or to whom you are talking. You depend on others for daily routines of getting dressed and being fed. Additionally, you are having great pain in your left hip. Hip replacement surgery could reduce pain and increase mobility. But there is no intervention without risk. Would you want to have the surgery? What are your arguments? Who should decide?

[Testing: S1.1—3; V2, 3, 7, 8; PES 1—4, 6, 12-15]

Expected response:

Actual response:

Physician's comment:

Physician's Concluding Evaluation

1. *Value Assessment*   (Date: Updated: Updated:)
   Clarity:
   Priorities:
   Issues undecided or unclear:

2. *Advance Directive*   (Date: Updated: Updated:)
   Clarity:
   Priorities:
   Issues undecided or unclear:
   Proxy Decision Maker(s) [name, phone, fax]:

SOURCE: From Rita Kielstein and Hans-Martin Sass. Using Stories to Assess Values and Establish Medical Directives. *Kennedy Institute of Ethics Journal*(3). Pp. 319-25. © 1993. The Johns Hopkins University Press. Reprinted with permission.

VALUES HISTORY (VH)

Developed by David J. Doukas and
Laurence B. McCullough

INSTRUMENT DEVELOPMENT, ADMINISTRATION, AND SCORING

The Values History (VH) serves as an adjunct to advance directives and can be used as a clinical and a research tool to elicit the values of the patient as these values pertain to chronic and critical medical care. The VH is to be used with competent patients to give the health care team a more complete understanding of the patient's preferences and directions. More specifically, the goal of this process is to help the patient become clear about what he or she wants or does not want and why, as well as to help health professionals and institutions to understand, respect, and implement the cluster of value-based decisions from the VH (Doukas & McCullough, 1991).

The VH has two parts: (a) an explicit identification of values and (b) the articulation of ADs based on the patient's values. After a patient has signed a living will and the "Values Section" of the VH is completed, the physician would begin the patient education and disclosure process that leads to discussion and possible signing of the "Directives Section"of the VH (Doukas & McCullough, 1991). The "Directives Section" includes items relevant to acute and long-term care. Each is initialed by the patient and dated as they are decided over time, and for each item the patient is asked to explain reasons and motivations.

In addition to its clinical use as an extension of the AD, the VH has been used as a research tool to study questions of cross-generation values (Doukas, Antonucci, & Gorenflo, 1992). For studies, a 1-to-7 (from negative to positive) Likert scale is used for values and a 1-to-5 (strongly agree to strongly disagree) for quality of life versus length-of-life statements or 1-to-5 (never implement to always implement) for medical interventions listed on the VH (Doukas & Gorenflo, 1993). Reilly, Teasdale, and McCullough (1994) used the interventions portion of the VH (rated as never, trial of therapy to assess efficacy, or always) with four scenarios (usual health, terminal illness, coma, or Alzheimer's disease) with 218 healthy, well-educated, largely Caucasian community dwellers aged 60 and older. The trial of therapy option was strongly favored. Mold, Looney, Viviani, and Quiggens (1994) have used a modified version of the VH to study preferences of 178 cognitively intact patients at a geriatric clinic. Although too limited to form norms, the findings do provide comparison for other populations. Quality of life rather than quantity of life and ability to think clearly rather than other health-related values were considered important by 82% of the subjects. Most considered persistent vegetative state (PVS) to be worse than death. Sociodemographic and functional status variables were weak predictors of personal values and directives, thereby supporting the significance of routinely eliciting patient values and preferences.

PSYCHOMETRIC PROPERTIES

The validity of the VH is based on the ethical consideration that it enhances autonomy of the patient by clarifying values and preferences in a way that present ADs do not. In pilot testing with patients, items in the "Values Section" are those that express commonly held values in patient health care decision making.

In a study of undergraduates, factor analysis showed the values domains of communication/autonomy (Cronbach's alpha = .69) and family pain/burden (Cronbach's alpha = .72) within the overall value domain. Within the overall directives domain, long-term care (Cronbach's alpha = .91) and basic-care scales (Cronbach's alpha = .86) were found (Doukas et al., 1992). When asked to assume they had a terminal illness, a study of 125 cognitively intact adult outpatients without terminal illness yielded three factors: communication issues (Cronbach's alpha = .69), family burden (Cronbach's alpha = .66), and physician compliance (Cronbach's alpha = .67) in the value domain. In the directive domain, factors of basic ongoing care such as medication and hydration, enteral feeding tubes (Cronbach's alpha = .80), fundamental-acute care including ICU (Cronbach's alpha = .76), and code-support factors (Cronbach's alpha = .87) were found. Significant correlations have been found between patient values and the medical therapies patients would wish to forego if they were terminally ill (Doukas & McCullough, 1995), supporting validity of the VH.

SUMMARY AND CRITIQUE

The Values History and similar methods have been criticized as being general and vague and not necessarily a suitable guide to deducing a patient's view on specific interventions. Because people's values are frequently inconsistent or in conflict with no clear resolution, the choices they would make in a particular clinical situation are not clear, which further complicates the matter. Processes described to establish content validity are vague and apparently did not employ commonly used methods for this purpose. No studies that tested use of the VH with patients who became terminally ill could be located. Populations studied appear to be ethnically and economically homogeneous, although there is reason to believe that preferences might be quite different across populations (Reilly et al., 1994). Sensitivity of the VH to interventions has apparently not been studied.

Although less relevant to its use as a measurement instrument, there may be instances in which state law required alterations of some portions of the VH (Doukas & McCullough, 1991). A finding that family burden is significant in a terminal care decision has emerged from research using the VH.

REFERENCES

Doukas, D. J., Antonucci, T., & Gorenflo, D. W. (1992). A multigenerational study on the correlation of values and advanced directives. *Ethics & Behavior, 2*, 51-59.

Doukas, D. J., & Gorenflo, D. W. (1993). Analyzing the values history: An evaluation of patient medical values and advance directives. *The Journal of Clinical Ethics, 4*, 41-45.

Doukas, D. J., & McCullough, L. B. (1991). The Values History. *The Journal of Family Practice, 32*, 145-153.

Doukas, D. J., & McCullough, L. B. (1995). The Values History in well elder care. In W. Reichel (Ed.), *Care of the elderly: Clinical aspects of aging* (4th ed.). Baltimore: Williams & Wilkins.

Mold, J. W., Looney, S. W., Viviani, N. J., & Quiggens, P. A. (1994). Predicting the health-related values and preferences of geriatric patients. *The Journal of Family Practice, 39*, 461-467.

Reilly, R. B., Teasdale, T. A., & McCullough, L. B. (1994). Projecting patients' preferences from living wills: An invalid strategy for management of dementia with life-threatening illness. *Journal of the American Geriatrics Society, 42*, 997-1003.

Instrument 5.2

THE VALUES HISTORY

Patient Name: _____

This Values History serves as a set of my specific value-based directives for various medical interventions. It is to be used in health care circumstances when I may be unable to voice my preferences. These directives shall be made a part of the medical record and used as supplementary to my living will and/or durable power of attorney for health care.

I. VALUES SECTION
There are several values important in decisions about terminal treatment and care. This section of the Values History invites you to identify your most important values.

A. Basic Life Values
Perhaps the most basic values in this context concern length of life versus quality of life. Which of the following two statements is the most important to you?

_____ 1. I want to live as long as possible, regardless of the quality of life that I experience.

_____ 2. I want to preserve a good quality of life, if this means that I may not live as long.

B. Quality of Life Values
There are many values that help us to define for ourselves the quality of life that we want to live. The following list contains some that appear to be very important. Review this list (and feel free either to elaborate on it, or to add to it) and circle those values that are most important to your definition of quality of life.

1. I want to maintain my capacity to think clearly.
2. I want to feel safe and secure.
3. I want to avoid unnecessary pain and suffering.
4. I want to be treated with respect.
5. I want to be treated with dignity when I can no longer speak for myself.
6. I do not want to be an unnecessary burden on my family.
7. I want to be able to make my own decisions.
8. I want to experience a comfortable dying process.
9. I want to be with my loved ones before I die.
10. I want to leave good memories of me to my loved ones.
11. I want to be treated in accord with my religious beliefs and traditions.
12. I want respect shown for my body after I die.
13. I want to help others by making a contribution to medical education and research.
14. Other values or clarification of values above:

II. DIRECTIVES SECTION

Some directives involve simple yes or no decisions. Others provide for the choice of a trial of intervention. Initials/Date

_____ 1. I want to undergo cardiopulmonary resuscitation.

       _____ TRIAL to determine effectiveness using reasonable medical judgment.

       _____ NO

       Why?

_____ 2. I want to be placed on a ventilator.

       _____ YES

       _____ TRIAL for the TIME PERIOD OF _____

       _____ TRIAL to determine effectiveness using reasonable medical judgment.

       _____ NO

       Why?

_____ 3. I want to have an endoctracheal tube used in order to perform items 1 and 2.

       _____ YES

       _____ TRIAL for the TIME PERIOD OF _____

       _____ TRIAL to determine effectiveness using reasonable medical judgment.

       _____ NO

       Why?

_____ 4. I want to have total parenteral nutrition administered for my nutrition.

       _____ YES

       _____ TRIAL for the TIME PERIOD OF _____

       _____ TRIAL to determine effectiveness using reasonable medical judgment.

       _____ NO

       Why?

_____ 5. I want to have intravenous medication and hydration administered; regardless of my decision, I understand that intravenous hydration to alleviate discomfort or pain medication will not be withheld from me if I so request them.

       _____ YES

       _____ TRIAL for the TIME PERIOD OF _____

       _____ TRIAL to determine effectiveness using reasonable medical judgment.

       _____ NO

       Why?

_____ 6. I want to have all medications used for the treatment of my illness continued; regardless of my decision, I understand that pain medication will continue to be administered including narcotic medications.

       _____ YES

       _____ TRIAL for the TIME PERIOD OF _____

       _____ TRIAL to determine effectiveness using reasonable medical judgment.

       _____ NO

       Why?

_____ 7. I want to have nasogastric, gastrostomy or other enteral feeding tubes introduced and administered for my nutrition.

      _____ YES

      _____ TRIAL for the TIME PERIOD OF _____

      _____ TRIAL to determine effectiveness using reasonable medical judgment.

      _____ NO

Why?

_____ 8. I want to be placed on a dialysis machine.

      _____ YES

      _____ TRIAL for the TIME PERIOD OF _____

      _____ TRIAL to determine effectiveness using reasonable medical judgment.

      _____ NO

Why?

_____ 9. I want to have an autopsy done to determine the cause(s) of my death.

      _____ YES

      _____ NO

Why?

_____10. I want to be admitted to the Intensive Care Unit for my medical care, if necessary.

      _____ YES

      _____ NO

Why?

_____11. *For patients in long-term care facilities or receiving care at home who experience a life-threatening change in health status:* I want 911 called in case of a medical emergency.

      _____ YES

      _____ NO

Why?

_____12. OTHER DIRECTIVES:

I consent to these directives after receiving honest disclosures of their implications, risks, and benefits by my physician, free from constraints and being of sound mind.

_____   _____

Signature   Date

_____

Witness

_____

Witness

13. PROXY NEGATION:

I request that the following persons NOT be allowed to make decisions on my behalf in the event of my disability or incapacity:

_____

_____

_____

_____   _____
Signature   Date

_____
Witness

_____
Witness

14. ORGAN DONATION:

   Specific State Version Inserted Here

15. DURABLE POWER OF ATTORNEY FOR HEALTH CARE:

   Specific State Version Inserted Here

SOURCE: © Appleton and Lange, Doukas, D. J., & McCullough, L. B. The Values History: The Evaluation of the Patient's Values and Advance Directives. *Journal of Family Practice*, 1991; 32(1):145-153. Reproduced with permission from The Journal of Family Practice.

ADVANCE DIRECTIVE-HIV QUESTIONNAIRE (AD-HIV)

Developed by Nitsa Kohut, Mehran Sam,
Keith O'Rourke, Douglas K. MacFadden,
Irving Salit, and Peter A. Singer

INSTRUMENT DEVELOPMENT, ADMINISTRATION, AND SCORING

Because the usefulness of advance directives depends on the stability of individuals' treatment preferences over time, it is important to understand conditions of stability. The effects of potentially reversible factors such as impaired physical function, depression, or lack of social support on treatment preferences are also key (Kohut et al., 1997).

The AD-HIV Questionnaire is a modification of Emanuel and Emanuel's Medical Directive (1989), reviewed elsewhere in this chapter. It elicits preferences for four life-sustaining treatments (CPR, mechanical ventilation, artificial nutrition, and hydration and antibiotics) in three scenarios of mental incompetence: irreversible cognitive impairment, reversible cognitive impairment with residual functional disability, and reversible cognitive impairment with full functional recovery. Each of the 12 possible choices is to be rated as "want" (0), "do not want" (1), or "undecided" (0). Values for the 12 choices are summed and divided by the number of nonmissing values, to create a summary score between 0 and 1. This summary score is an overall estimate of a patient's refusal of life-sustaining treatment (Kohut et al., 1997).

In the scenario with the best prognosis (reversible with full functional recovery), most participants wanted life-sustaining treatment; in the scenario with the worst prognosis (irreversible), most did not. The scenario had a stronger influence on a person's preferences than did the treatment. Treatment preferences were unstable. In six months, 80% of participants changed at least one treatment choice, and 50% changed from wanting to not wanting treatment, or vice versa (Kohut et al., 1997).

PSYCHOMETRIC PROPERTIES

The AD-HIV was reviewed for face and content validity by six clinicians who cared for people living with HIV. The life-sustaining treatments used in those situations were judged to be common scenarios of incompetency for patients in the HIV population. In a pilot study, patients rated the desirability of the scenarios in the order one would expect (i.e., reversible cognitive impairment with full recovery, reversible cognitive impairment with residual functional disability, and irreversible cognitive impairment). This finding provides some support for construct validity (Kohut et al., 1997).

The AD-HIV was tested with a convenience sample of 150 HIV-positive patients attending an outpatient clinic. To evaluate test-retest reliability, a subset of participants was asked to complete a second AD-HIV questionnaire within five days; over this span only 23 of 63 patients had not changed in their preferences in any of the three scenarios. A total of 112 changes (out of a possible 744) were observed. "Norms" established by this group showed that in the reversible scenarios, 65% to 90% of participants wanted life-sustaining treatment; in the irreversible scenario, 9% to 48% wanted life-sustaining treatment (Kohut, 1993).

SUMMARY AND CRITIQUE

The findings of the single study using the AD-HIV suggest that because most changed some of their preferences, people should update their ADs at regular intervals. Kohut et al. do note imperfect test-retest reliability characteristics over even a very brief time (five days). In addition, evidence supporting content and construct validity is currently limited.

REFERENCES

Emanuel, L. L., & Emanuel, E. J. (1989). The Medical Directive. *Journal of the American Medical Association, 261,* 3288-3293.

Kohut, N. (1993). *Preference for life-sustaining treatment of patients with HIV-related disease.* Unpublished master's thesis, University of Toronto.

Kohut, N., Sam, M., O'Rourke, K., MacFadden, D. K., Salit, I., & Singer, P. A. (1997). Stability of treatment preferences: Although most preferences do not change, most people change some of their preferences. *The Journal of Clinical Ethics, 8,* 124-135.

Instrument 5.3

AD-HIV QUESTIONNAIRE

The advance directive questionnaire describes three hypothetical situations in which you would be too ill to participate in the making of decisions about your medical care. In each situation you will be asked about four different life-sustaining treatments that you may want, not want, or are undecided about.

The life-sustaining treatments involved are:

1. **Cardiopulmonary resuscitation (CPR):**
   This is used to restart your heart. It involves chest compressions, artificial breathing by placing a tube down the throat, electric shock to the heart, and various drugs.

2. **Mechanical breathing:**
   This is used when you cannot breathe on your own. It involves placing a tube down the throat, and hooking it up to a machine that breathes for you. You are unable to talk and eat while you are hooked up to the machine.

3. **Artificial nutrition and hydration:**
   This is used when you cannot eat or drink by mouth. A tube is placed in the stomach or in the vein and fluids and nutrition are given through this tube.

4. **Antibiotics:**
   These are drugs used to treat infection and are usually given through a tube placed in the vein.

Situation A

Suppose you were to develop an *irreversible* illness that made you *permanently* unable to make decisions or communicate meaningfully. You could not remember things, think clearly, or recognize people. You would also not be able to take care of yourself and would need help bathing, eating, and going to the bathroom.

If you were in this situation, and a life-threatening problem arose, what would your wishes be regarding the use of the following life-sustaining treatments?

Assume that if you receive the treatment you would continue to live in the situation described; if you did not receive the treatment, you would likely die.

Please check one box for each treatment.

	I Want	I Do Not Want	I Am Undecided
Cardiopulmonary resuscitation: The use of drugs, electric shocks, and chest compressions to restart the heart			
Mechanical breathing: Breathing by machine			
Artificial nutrition and hydration: Fluids and nutrition given through a tube			
Antibiotics: Drugs to treat infection			

Situation B

Suppose you were to develop a *reversible* illness that made you *temporarily* unable to make decisions or communicate meaningfully. You would likely recover from this illness and would be able to return home and care for yourself.

If you were in this situation, and a life-threatening problem arose, what would your wishes be regarding the use of the following life-sustaining treatments?

Assume that if you did receive the treatment you would continue to live in the described situation; if you did not receive the treatment, you would likely die.

Please check one box for each treatment.

	I Want	I Do Not Want	I Am Undecided
Cardiopulmonary resuscitation: The use of drugs, electric shocks, and chest compressions to restart the heart			
Mechanical breathing: Breathing by machine			
Artificial nutrition and hydration: Fluids and nutrition given through a tube			
Antibiotics: Drugs to treat infection			

Situation C

Suppose you were to develop a *reversible* illness that made you *temporarily* unable to make decisions or communicate meaningfully. You would likely recover from this illness but you would not be able to live at home alone or take care of yourself. You would need help bathing, eating, and going to the bathroom.

If you were in this situation, and a life-threatening problem arose, what would your wishes be regarding the use of the following life-sustaining treatments?

Assume that if you did receive the treatment you would continue to live in the described situation; if you did not receive the treatment, you would likely die.

Please check one box for each treatment.

	I Want	I Do Not Want	I Am Undecided
Cardiopulmonary resuscitation: The use of drugs, electric shocks, and chest compressions to restart the heart			
Mechanical breathing: Breathing by machine			
Artificial nutrition and hydration: Fluids and nutrition given through a tube			
Antibiotics: Drugs to treat infection			

SOURCE: From "Stability of treatment preferences: Although most preferences do not change, most people change some of their preferences," by N. Kohut, M. Sam, K. O'Rourke, D. K. MacFadden, I. Salit, and P. A. Singer, 1997, *Journal of Clinical Ethics, 8,* pp. 124-135. Copyright 1997 by The Journal of Clinical Ethics. All rights reserved. Reprinted with permission from *Journal of Clinical Ethics.*

THE MEDICAL DIRECTIVE (MD)

Developed by Linda L. Emanuel
and Ezekiel J. Emanuel

INSTRUMENT DEVELOPMENT, ADMINISTRATION, AND SCORING

Predrafted advance directives (ADs) can be structured as clinical assessment instruments that explore an individual's wishes and how these wishes reflect a particular view of life and the process of dying. The Medical Directive (MD) provides four paradigmatic scenarios (coma with a chance of recovery, persistent vegetative state, dementia, and dementia with terminal illness) that encompass the spectrum of incompetence. They also represent the principal circumstances arising in medical practice that have prompted legal cases. The MD also includes 11 medical interventions commonly employed for diagnosis and treatment of incompetent patients, four options (want, don't want, undecided, want trial), as well as other advance planning decisions such as proxy and organ donation. The patient provides information about choices, thus describing a pattern of preferences with a level of detail that should make interpretation clearer than in other AD formats.

The MD has been studied with 405 outpatients and 102 members of the general public. Completing the MD took an average of 14 minutes (Emanuel, Barry, Stoeckle, Ettelson, & Emanuel, 1991).

PSYCHOMETRIC PROPERTIES

Validity and reliability of the MD have been much more extensively studied than have most measurement tools in clinical ethics. Indeed, the concept of an AD as a clinical and research assessment tool is relatively novel. Few predrafted forms for advance care planning have been designed and tested against standards of reliability and validity (Alpert, Hoijtink, Fischer, & Emanuel, 1996). Reliability (internal consistency) coefficients were .98 for outpatients, .93 for the public, and .97 for physicians.

The illness circumstances depicted in the scenarios were chosen for their paradigmatic nature for disability and prognosis, types of mental incompetence, and the kinds of circumstances that have prompted legal cases, as well as the typical range of diagnostic and therapeutic interventions and patient decisions (Emanuel & Emanuel, 1989).

Emanuel and Emanuel cite as evidence of criterion validity the finding that results from the MD could be seen as a pattern of moral reasoning that could be used to infer other choices specified by the same patients (Alpert et al., 1996; Emanuel, Barry, Emanuel, & Stoeckle, 1994). Such evidence is important because application of stated preferences to eventual circumstances has been a problematic element of ADs.

Construct validity of an instrument depends on the existence of logical relationships among its measures and between its measures and higher order concepts. In the case of the MD, this requires looking for sensible relationships between treatment preferences, scenarios, and goals for care (Alpert et al., 1996). Construct validity for the MD is supported with findings of decreasing receptiveness to treatment with increasing severity of the illnesses described. In addition, less invasive treatments were accepted more often than more invasive treatments among subjects who differentiated between treatments (Alpert et al., 1996). Emanuel, Barry, et al. (1994) showed that these treatment choices also predicted unspecified decisions following considerations of prognosis and treatment invasiveness (criterion validity). Predictions for interventions of similar invasiveness were only in the intermediate range of predictive power, as were extrapolation of a patient's wishes across scenarios (predictive validity) (Emanuel & Emanuel, 1989).

The common assumption justifying the use of ADs is that a patient's prior expression of treatment choice accurately represents his or her future choices (i.e., they are stable over time). The stability of

MDs through 12 months (κ = .35) showed 72% agreement, which was highest among patients who had discussions with their physicians and among those with more education. Although patients showed a wide range of stability, those starting out stable rarely became less so (Emanuel, Emanuel, et al., 1994). That people decided against life-sustaining treatments about 70% of the time when imagining themselves incompetent with a poor prognosis is a point of comparison for other populations (Emanuel et al., 1991).

SUMMARY AND CRITIQUE

A major concern with ADs has been their ability to anticipate the exact circumstances that may eventually arise, fulfilling their role of extending patients' autonomy into times of incompetence. As well as being a form of AD, the MD may be used as a research tool to study physicians' and patients' attitudes and decisions about life-sustaining treatment (Alpert et al., 1996). It provides a structure of clinical circumstances, interventions, options, and goals to which patients can respond (Emanuel & Emanuel, 1989).

Use of a number of scenarios and treatment beyond the usual resuscitation and mechanical ventilation decisions increases the predictive validity of the MD. Thus, from a partial directive, a probability that a patient would have declined a particular intervention can be predicted. The range of predictive power was higher in extrapolation of individual patients' autonomous prior decisions than that of proxy decision making (Emanuel, Barry, et al., 1994).

The MD is one modality of preference expression. It should be further tested with different patient cohorts. In addition, its sensitivity to interventions such as discussion of or education about preferences must be established. Studies of the MD asked people to imagine themselves in these scenarios. No studies that compared the previously imagined responses to responses to similar actual circumstances could be located. Furthermore, stability data were not collected from patients who needed life-sustaining treatment. Other studies have found that these individuals may change their minds more often (Emanuel, Emanuel, et al., 1994).

REFERENCES

Alpert, H. R., Hoijtink, H., Fischer, G. S., & Emanuel, L. (1996). Psychometric analysis of an advance directive. *Medical Care, 34,* 1057-1065.

Emanuel, L. L., Barry, M. J., Emanuel, E. J., & Stoeckle, J. D. (1994). Advance directives: Can patients' stated treatment choices be used to infer unstated choices? *Medical Care, 32,* 95-105.

Emanuel, L. L., Barry, M. J., Stoeckle, J. D., Ettelson, L. M., & Emanuel, E. J. (1991). Advance directives for medical care—a case for greater use. *New England Journal of Medicine, 324,* 889-895.

Emanuel, L. L., & Emanuel, E. J. (1989). The Medical Directive. *Journal of the American Medical Association, 261,* 3288-3293.

Emanuel, L. L., Emanuel, E. J., Stoeckle, J. D., Hummel, L. R., & Barry, M. J. (1994). Advance directives: Stability of patients' treatment choices. *Archives of Internal Medicine, 154,* 209-217.

Instrument 5.4

THE MEDICAL DIRECTIVE

Introduction. As part of a person's right to self-determination, every adult may accept or refuse any recommended medical treatment. This is relatively easy when people are well and can speak. Unfortunately, during serious illness they are often unconscious or otherwise unable to communicate their wishes—at the very time when many critical decisions need to be made.

The Medical Directive allows you to record your wishes regarding various types of medical treatments in several representative situations so that your desires can be respected. It also lets you appoint a proxy, someone to make medical decisions in your place if you should become unable to make them on your own.

The Medical Directive comes into effect only if you become incompetent (unable to make decisions and too sick to have wishes). You can change it at any time until then. As long as you are competent, you should discuss your care directly with your physician.

Completing the form. You should, if possible complete the form in the context of a discussion with your physician. Ideally, this should occur in the presence of your proxy. This lets your physician and your proxy know how you think about these decisions, and it provides you and your physician with the opportunity to give or clarify relevant personal or medical information. You may also wish to discuss the issues with your family, friends, or religious mentor.

The Medical Directive contains six illness situations that include incompetence. For each one, you consider possible interventions and goals of medical care. Situation A is permanent coma; B is near death; C is with weeks to live in and out of consciousness; D is extreme dementia; E is a situation you describe; and F is temporary inability to make decisions.

For each scenario you identify your general goals for care and specific intervention choices. The interventions are divided into six groups: 1) cardiopulmonary resuscitation or major surgery; 2) mechanical breathing or dialysis; 3) blood transfusions or blood products; 4) artificial nutrition and hydration; 5) simple diagnostic tests or antibiotics; and 6) pain medications, even if they dull consciousness and indirectly shorten life. Most of these treatments are described briefly. If you have further questions, consult your physician.

Your wishes for treatment options (I want this treatment; I want this treatment tried, but stopped if there is no clear improvement; I am undecided; I do not want this treatment) should be indicated. If you choose a trial of treatment, you should understand that this indicates you want the treatment *withdrawn* if your physician and proxy believe that it has become futile.

The Personal Statement section allows you to explain your choices, and say anything you wish to those who may make decisions for you concerning the limits of your life and the goals of intervention. For example, in situation B, if you wish to define "uncertain chance" with numerical probability, you may do so here.

Next you may express your preferences concerning organ donation. Do you wish to donate your body or some or all of your organs after your death? If so, for what purpose(s) and to which physician or institution? If not, this should also be indicated in the appropriate box.

In the final section you may designate one or more proxies, who would be asked to make choices under circumstances in which your wishes are unclear. You can indicate whether or not the decisions of the proxy should override your wishes if there are differences. And, should you name more than one proxy, you can state who is to have the final say if there is disagreement. Your proxy must understand that this role usually involves making judgments that you would have made for yourself, had you been able—and making them by the criteria you have outlined. Proxy decisions should ideally be made in discussion with your family, friends, and physician.

What to do with the form. Once you have completed the form, you and two adult witnesses (other than your proxy) who have no interest in your estate need to sign and date it.

Many states have legislation covering documents of this sort. To determine the laws in your state, you should call the state attorney general's office or consult a lawyer. If your state has a statutory document, you may wish to use the Medical Directive and append it to this form.

You should give a copy of the completed document to your physician. His or her signature is desirable but not mandatory. The Directive should be placed in your medical records and flagged so that anyone who might be involved in your care can be aware of its presence. Your proxy, a family member, and/or a friend should also have a copy. In addition, you may want to carry a wallet card noting that you have such a document and where it can be found.

MY MEDICAL DIRECTIVE

This Medical Directive shall stand as a guide to my wishes regarding medical treatments in the event that illness should make me unable to communicate them directly. I make this Directive, being 18 years or more of age, of sound mind, and appreciating the consequences of my decisions.

SITUATION A

If I am in a coma or a persistent vegetative state and, in the opinion of my physician and two consultants, have no known hope of regaining awareness and higher mental functions no matter what is done, then my goals and specific wishes—if medically reasonable—for this and any additional illness would be:

[ ] prolong life; treat everything
[ ] attempt to cure, but reevaluate often
[ ] limit to less invasive and less burdensome interventions
[ ] provide comfort care only
[ ] other (*please specify*): _____

_____

Please check appropriate boxes:	I want	I want treatment tried. If no clear improvement, stop.	I am undecided	I do not want
1. Cardiopulmonary resuscitation (chest compressions, drugs, electric shocks, and artificial breathing aimed at reviving a person who is on the point of dying).		*Not applicable*		
2. Major surgery (for example, removing the gallbladder or part of the colon).		*Not applicable*		
3. Mechanical breathing (respiration by machine, through a tube in the throat).				
4. Dialysis (cleaning the blood by machine or by fluid passed through the belly).				
5. Blood transfusions or blood products.		*Not applicable*		
6. Artificial nutrition and hydration (given through a tube in a vein or in the stomach).				
7. Simple diagnostic tests (for example, blood tests or x-rays).		*Not applicable*		
8. Antibiotics (drugs used to fight infection).		*Not applicable*		
9. Pain medications, even if they dull consciousness and indirectly shorten my life.		*Not applicable*		

SITUATION B

If I am near death and in a coma and, in the opinion of my physician and two consultants, have a small but uncertain chance of regaining higher mental functions, a somewhat greater chance of surviving with permanent mental and physical disability, and a much greater chance of not recovering at all, then my goals and specific wishes—if medically reasonable—for this and any additional illness would be:

[ ] prolong life; treat everything
[ ] attempt to cure, but reevaluate often
[ ] limit to less invasive and less burdensome interventions
[ ] provide comfort care only
[ ] other (*please specify*): _____

_____

Please check appropriate boxes:	I want	I want treatment tried. If no clear improvement, stop.	I am undecided	I do not want
1. Cardiopulmonary resuscitation (chest compressions, drugs, electric shocks, and artificial breathing aimed at reviving a person who is on the point of dying).		*Not applicable*		
2. Major surgery (for example, removing the gallbladder or part of the colon).		*Not applicable*		
3. Mechanical breathing (respiration by machine, through a tube in the throat).				
4. Dialysis (cleaning the blood by machine or by fluid passed through the belly).				
5. Blood transfusions or blood products.		*Not applicable*		

6. Artificial nutrition and hydration (given through a tube in a vein or in the stomach).			
7. Simple diagnostic tests (for example, blood tests or x-rays).	*Not applicable*		
8. Antibiotics (drugs used to fight infection).	*Not applicable*		
9. Pain medications, even if they dull consciousness and indirectly shorten my life.	*Not applicable*		

SITUATION C

If I have a terminal illness with weeks to live, and my mind is not working well enough to make decisions for myself, but I am sometimes awake and seem to have feelings, then my goals and specific wishes—if medically reasonable—for this and any additional illness would be:

*In this state, prior wishes need to be balanced with a best guess about your current feelings. The proxy and physician have to make this judgment for you.

[ ] prolong life; treat everything
[ ] attempt to cure, but reevaluate often
[ ] limit to less invasive and less burdensome interventions
[ ] provide comfort care only
[ ] other (*please specify*): _____
_____

Please check appropriate boxes:	I want	I want treatment tried. If no clear improvement, stop.	I am undecided	I do not want
1. Cardiopulmonary resuscitation (chest compressions, drugs, electric shocks, and artificial breathing aimed at reviving a person who is on the point of dying).		*Not applicable*		
2. Major surgery (for example, removing the gallbladder or part of the colon).		*Not applicable*		
3. Mechanical breathing (respiration by machine, through a tube in the throat).				
4. Dialysis (cleaning the blood by machine or by fluid passed through the belly).				
5. Blood transfusions or blood products.		*Not applicable*		
6. Artificial nutrition and hydration (given through a tube in a vein or in the stomach).				
7. Simple diagnostic tests (for example, blood tests or x-rays).		*Not applicable*		
8. Antibiotics (drugs used to fight infection).		*Not applicable*		
9. Pain medications, even if they dull consciousness and indirectly shorten my life.		*Not applicable*		

SITUATION D

If I have brain damage or some brain disease that in the opinion of my physician and two consultants cannot be reversed and that makes me unable to think or have feelings, *but I have no terminal illness,* then my goals and specific wishes—if medically reasonable—for this and any additional illness would be:

[ ] prolong life; treat everything
[ ] attempt to cure, but reevaluate often
[ ] limit to less invasive and less burdensome interventions
[ ] provide comfort care only
[ ] other (*please specify*): _____

Please check appropriate boxes:	I want	I want treatment tried. If no clear improvement, stop.	I am undecided	I do not want
1. Cardiopulmonary resuscitation (chest compressions, drugs, electric shocks, and artificial breathing aimed at reviving a person who is on the point of dying).		*Not applicable*		
2. Major surgery (for example, removing the gallbladder or part of the colon).		*Not applicable*		
3. Mechanical breathing (respiration by machine, through a tube in the throat).				
4. Dialysis (cleaning the blood by machine or by fluid passed through the belly).				
5. Blood transfusions or blood products.		*Not applicable*		
6. Artificial nutrition and hydration (given through a tube in a vein or in the stomach).				

		I want treatment tried. If no clear improvement, stop.		
7. Simple diagnostic tests (for example, blood tests or x-rays).		*Not applicable*		
8. Antibiotics (drugs used to fight infection).		*Not applicable*		
9. Pain medications, even if they dull consciousness and indirectly shorten my life.		*Not applicable*		

SITUATION E

If I . . .

(describe a situation that is important to you and/or your doctor believes you should consider in view of your current medical situation):

[ ] prolong life; treat everything
[ ] attempt to cure, but reevaluate often
[ ] limit to less invasive and less burdensome interventions
[ ] provide comfort care only
[ ] other (*please specify*): _____

_____

Please check appropriate boxes:	I want	I want treatment tried. If no clear improvement, stop.	I am undecided	I do not want
1. Cardiopulmonary resuscitation (chest compressions, drugs, electric shocks, and artificial breathing aimed at reviving a person who is on the point of dying).		*Not applicable*		
2. Major surgery (for example, removing the gallbladder or part of the colon).		*Not applicable*		

3. Mechanical breathing (respiration by machine, through a tube in the throat).				
4. Dialysis (cleaning the blood by machine or by fluid passed through the belly).				
5. Blood transfusions or blood products.	*Not applicable*			
6. Artificial nutrition and hydration (given through a tube in a vein or in the stomach).				
7. Simple diagnostic tests (for example, blood tests or x-rays).	*Not applicable*			
8. Antibiotics (drugs used to fight infection).	*Not applicable*			
9. Pain medications, even if they dull consciousness and indirectly shorten my life.	*Not applicable*			

SITUATION F

If I am in my current state of health (describe briefly):_____

_____

_____

and then have an illness that, in the opinion of my physician and two consultants, is life threatening but reversible, and I am temporarily unable to make decisions, then my goals and specific wishes—if medically reasonable—would be:

[ ] prolong life; treat everything

[ ] attempt to cure, but reevaluate often

[ ] limit to less invasive and less burdensome interventions

[ ] provide comfort care only

[ ] other *(please specify)*: _____

_____

_____

Please check appropriate boxes:	I want	I want treatment tried. If no clear improve-ment, stop.	I am un-decided	I do not want
1. Cardiopulmonary resuscitation (chest compressions, drugs, electric shocks, and artificial breathing aimed at reviving a person who is on the point of dying).		*Not applicable*		
2. Major surgery (for example, removing the gallbladder or part of the colon).		*Not applicable*		
3. Mechanical breathing (respiration by machine, through a tube in the throat).				
4. Dialysis (cleaning the blood by machine or by fluid passed through the belly).				
5. Blood transfusions or blood products.		*Not applicable*		
6. Artificial nutrition and hydration (given through a tube in a vein or in the stomach).				
7. Simple diagnostic tests (for example, blood tests or x-rays).		*Not applicable*		
8. Antibiotics (drugs used to fight infection).		*Not applicable*		
9. Pain medications, even if they dull consciousness and indirectly shorten my life.		*Not applicable*		

HEALTH CARE PROXY

I appoint as my proxy decision-maker(s):

_____
Name and Address

and *(optional)*

_____
Name and Address

I direct my proxy to make health-care decisions based on his/her assessment of my personal wishes. If my personal desires are unknown, my proxy is to make health-care decisions based on his/her best guess as to my wishes. My proxy shall have the authority to make all health-care decisions for me, including decisions about life-sustaining treatment, if I am unable to make them myself. My proxy's authority becomes effective if my attending physician determines in writing that I lack the capacity to make or to communicate health-care decisions. My proxy is then to have the same authority to make health-care decisions as I would if I had the capacity to make them, EXCEPT *(list the limitations, if any, you wish to place on your proxy's authority):*

I wish my written preference to be applied as exactly as possible/with flexibility according to my proxy's judgment. *(Delete as appropriate)*

Should there be any disagreement between the wishes I have indicated in this document and the decisions favored by my above-named proxy, I wish my proxy to have authority over my written statements/I wish my written statements to bind my proxy. *(Delete as appropriate)*

If I have appointed more than one proxy and there is disagreement between their wishes, _____ shall have final authority.

Signed: _____
         Signature   Printed Name

         _____
         Address   Date

Witness: _____
         Signature   Printed Name

         _____
         Address   Date

Witness: _____
         Signature   Printed Name

         _____

Address   Date

Physician *(optional):*

I am _____'s physician. I have seen this advance care document and have had an opportunity to discuss his/her preferences regarding medical interventions at the end of life. If _____ becomes incompetent, I understand that it is my duty to interpret and implement the preferences contained in this document in order to fulfill his/her wishes.

Signed: _____

       Signature   Printed Name

_____

       Address   Date

SOURCE: Copyright 1990 by Linda L. Emanuel and Ezekiel J. Emanuel. The authors of this form advise that it should be completed pursuant to a discussion between the principal and his or her physician, so that the principal can be adequately informed of any personal medical information, and so that the physician can be appraised of the intentions of the principal and the existence of such a document which may be made a part of the principal's medical records.

This form was originally published as part of an article by Linda L. Emanuel and Ezekiel J. Emanuel, "The Medical Directive: A New Comprehensive Advance Care Document" in *Journal of the American Medical Association,* June 9, 1989:261:3290. It does not reflect the official policy of the American Medical Association.

Copies of this form may be obtained from: The Medical Directive, P.O. Box 6100, Holliston, MA 01746-6100, 1-800-214-4553.

ADVANCE DIRECTIVE ACCEPTABILITY QUESTIONNAIRE (ADAQ)

Developed by Peter A. Singer, Elaine C. Thiel, C. David Naylor,
Robert M. A. Richardson, Hilary Llewellyn-Thomas,
Marc Goldstein, Carl Saiphoo, P. Robert Uldall,
Donald Kim, and David C. Mendelssohn

INSTRUMENT DEVELOPMENT, ADMINISTRATION, AND SCORING

An advance directive (AD) allows people to express what life-sustaining treatments they want (instruction directive) and who they want making these decisions for them (proxy directive). ADs are completed by capable individuals and become effective if and when they become incapable. Many public policy initiatives encourage their use (Reinders & Singer, 1994).

A variety of generic and disease-specific ADs exist, different in format, background information provided, and taxonomy and description of health states and treatments. The Advance Directive Acceptability Questionnaire (ADAQ) offers a set of criteria by which individuals can rate the acceptability of various ADs. This is useful for studying preferences for format and content of ADs and for instructing public policy and clinical practice about the availability of various ADs (Reinders & Singer, 1994).

Some background about disease-specific ADs may be helpful. It is very difficult to provide meaningful prognostic data in an AD that is intended for completion by patients with a wide variety of health problems. In addition, generic ADs must offer a large number of choices for an individual to consider, and that person will never confront most of these scenarios. Disease-specific ADs differ from generic ADs principally in the instruction component; they offer decisions faced by people with that disease. For example, an AD for patients with chronic obstructive pulmonary disease (COPD) focuses on whether to accept intubation and ventilation for acute respiratory failure, which is the prime decision these individuals will face. The limitation in number of decisions and the more precise prognostic data that can be provided makes understanding treatment options easier. Because the person already has experience with the illness that leads to these circumstances, the choices themselves are less hypothetical (Singer, 1994).

A copy of the Dialysis Living Will may be found in Mendelssohn and Singer (1994). It contains a greatly simplified instruction directive with only two treatment decisions—whether or not to commence CPR and whether or not to continue renal replacement therapy with dialysis. Empirical research aimed at evaluating and comparing the many available ADs will be necessary to determine which features lead a person to prefer one over another, and which best ensures that wishes are in fact followed as the patient's condition deteriorates (Mendelssohn & Singer, 1994).

The 13 items in the ADAQ are rated on a 5-point ordinal scale from poor = 0, fair = 1, good = 2, very good = 3, and excellent = 4. The total score is calculated by the addition of scores on each individual item, division by the highest possible score, and multiplication by 100, yielding a percent value.

The ADAQ could also be useful in the process of developing new ADs. This process should include study of face and content validity, pilot testing with individuals from the target audience of users, and estimate of reliability and other forms of validity such as fewer people choosing continuation of treatment as health states become more disabling (Mendelssohn & Singer, 1994). If ADAQ had been broadly established for populations and disease entities, this instrument could be part of a standard of acceptability.

PSYCHOMETRIC PROPERTIES

Ninety-five adult patients receiving hemodialysis in 6 units in Toronto participated in the study that developed and tested the

ADAQ. Acceptability of three ADs were studied; all three combined proxy and instruction directives. Mean ADAQ scores for each AD were: Dialysis Living Will 71%, Centre for Bioethics Living Will 70%, and Medical Directive 60%.

The ADAQ was evaluated for content validity by an interdisciplinary panel. Internal consistency reliability coefficient (Cronbach's alpha) for the ADAQ was .93 (Singer et al., 1995).

SUMMARY AND CRITIQUE

Although ADAQ is itself a generic instrument, evidence of its use has thus far been reported only with people with dialysis in one metropolitan area. Its validity for various cultural groups and individuals in situations other than dialysis remain to be determined. Because dialysis patients have long-term relationships with their professional caregivers and are likely to experience clinical situations where ADs are of use, findings from the initial study may not be generalizable to other groups.

More formal study of ADAQ content validity for a variety of populations would be helpful.

REFERENCES

Mendelssohn, D. C., & Singer, P. A. (1994). Advance directives in dialysis. *Advances in Renal Replacement Therapy, 1,* 240-250.

Reinders, M., & Singer, P. A. (1994). Which advance directive do patients prefer? *Journal of General Internal Medicine, 9,* 49-51.

Singer, P. A. (1994). Disease-specific advance directives. *The Lancet, 344,* 594-596.

Singer, P. A., Thiel, E. C., Naylor, D., Richardson, R. M. A., Llewellyn-Thomas, H., Goldstein, M., Saiphoo, C., Uldall, P. R., Kim, D., & Mendelssohn, D. C. (1995). Life-sustaining treatment preferences of hemodialysis patients: Implications for advance directives. *Journal of the American Society of Nephrology, 6,* 1410-1417.

Instrument 5.5

Study _____   Subject ID [ ] [ ] [ ] [ ] [ ]

ADVANCE DIRECTIVE ACCEPTABILITY QUESTIONNAIRE

*This questionnaire asks about the living will (advance directive) you have just
completed. Please answer each question by circling the appropriate response.
There are no right or wrong answers. We are only interested in your opinion.*

HOW WOULD YOU RATE:	Excellent	Very good	Good	Fair	Poor	Don't know
The general information about living wills provided in this living will?	1	2	3	4	5	6
The simplicity of the language used in this living will?	1	2	3	4	5	6
The amount of detail in this living will?	1	2	3	4	5	6
The length of this living will?	1	2	3	4	5	6
The design or layout of this living will?	1	2	3	4	5	6
The description of situations in this living will?	1	2	3	4	5	6
The description of treatments in this living will?	1	2	3	4	5	6
How easy it was to give instructions about treatments?	1	2	3	4	5	6
How easy it was to appoint your proxy?	1	2	3	4	5	6
The way this living will raised potentially disturbing issues?	1	2	3	4	5	6
How well this living will allowed you to express your wishes?	1	2	3	4	5	6
How well this living will would give you control over your future medical care?	1	2	3	4	5	6
This living will overall?	1	2	3	4	5	6

Would you use this living will?

[ ] Yes—Why?

[ ] No—Why not?

How would you improve this living will?

Thank You

SOURCE: From "Life-sustaining treatment preferences of hemodialysis patients: Implications for advance directives," by P. A. Singer, E. C. Thiel, D. Naylor, R. M. A. Richardson, H. Llewellyn-Thomas, M. Goldstein, C. Saiphoo, P. R. Uldall, D. Kim, and D. C. Mendelssohn, 1995, *Journal of the American Society of Nephrology, 6*, pp. 1410-1417. Reprinted with permission.

ADVANCE DIRECTIVES QUESTIONNAIRE (ADQ)

*Developed by John E. Heffner, Bonnie Fahy,
Lana Hilling, and Celia Barbieri*

INSTRUMENT DEVELOPMENT, ADMINISTRATION, AND SCORING

Patients with chronic obstructive pulmonary disease and their families often face decisions about accepting life-support interventions at the terminal stages of their disease. Therefore, timely completion of ADs and patient-physician discussion about end-of-life issues are essential elements in preserving patient autonomy in health care decisions. Previous research has shown that only a minority of patients (those with moderate to severe lung dysfunction enrolled in pulmonary rehabilitation programs) have completed these steps and believe that their physicians understand their end-of-life support preferences. Although pulmonary rehabilitation programs may be effective sites for educating patients about the importance of ADs, only a minority do so (Heffner, Fahy, Hilling, & Barbieri, 1997).

The Advance Directives Questionnaire (ADQ) was developed to assess opinions toward end-of-life decision making of patients with chronic lung disease. It queries patients regarding demographic information, functional capacity, understanding and completion of ADs, participation with their physicians in decisions regarding end-of-life issues, and experience with previous hospitalizations and life-support interventions. Scoring procedures for the entire ADQ are not described. Responses to open-ended questions were coded into general categories (Heffner et al., 1997).

PSYCHOMETRIC PROPERTIES

The ADQ was tested with a group of elderly hospital volunteers to refine its clarity of language and readability. Test-retest reliability over a period of seven days was 90%. Heffner et al. indicate high construct validity, shown by complete concordance with an oral interview regarding responses to the questionnaire items. The ADQ was next administered to 93 patients with chronic obstructive lung disease—43 in a control group and 50 receiving an educational intervention on the importance of ADs. Most of the study outcomes were more likely in the educational group (Heffner et al., 1997), which could support sensitivity of the instrument to intervention.

SUMMARY AND CRITIQUE

Procedures by which content and construct validity were supported are incompletely described. Beginning psychometric work should be extended as should work on scoring.

REFERENCE

Heffner, J. E., Fahy, B., Hilling, L., & Barbieri, C. (1997). Outcomes of advance directive education of pulmonary rehabilitation patients. *American Journal of Respiratory and Critical Care Medicine, 155,* 1055-1059.

Instrument 5.6

Date_____   Patient #_____

ADVANCE DIRECTIVES QUESTIONNAIRE PART I

The Pulmonary Rehabilitation Program provides an opportunity to gather important information that allows us to develop a comprehensive care plan for your lung condition. One aspect of care important for all of us—both for patients with and without underlying chronic medical conditions—pertains to the preparation of Advance Directives. Advance Directives are written instruments that communicate our decisions regarding medical care in the event that a serious illness no longer allows us to voice our wishes, decisions, and opinions directly. In these circumstances, Advance Directives allow family members or friends, appointed in advance by ourselves, to watch over our well-being.

The following questionnaire will inventory your thoughts regarding Advance Directives. This information will assist us in designing our Pulmonary Rehabilitation Program in a manner that best suits your needs. Please answer all of the questions completely and ask us any questions if some portions of the questionnaire appear unclear.

Married [ ] Divorced [ ] Widowed [ ] Never married [ ]

Present and previous occupations _____
_____

1. Do you use oxygen at home?

    [ ] Yes
    [ ] No If NO is answered, skip to question number 4

2. If you DO use oxygen at home, what flow rate do you use?

    [ ] 1 L/min by nasal cannula
    [ ] 2 L/min by nasal cannula
    [ ] More than 2 L/min by nasal cannula
    [ ] Other _____

3. If you DO use oxygen at home, how many hours a day do you use it?

    [ ] Less than 12 hours a day
    [ ] More than 12 hours a day but less than 18 hours a day
    [ ] 18 to 24 hours a day

4. Is this your first time in Pulmonary Rehabilitation

   [ ] Yes

   [ ] No

> If No is answered, how many Pulmonary Rehabilitation Programs have you participated in *before* this one?

   [ ] One

   [ ] Two

   [ ] Three

5. How long have you participated in *this* Pulmonary Rehabilitation Program? _____(yrs/weeks/days)

6. What is your underlying lung condition? _____

_____

7. When you think of your lung condition, what worries or concerns come to mind? _____

_____

8. Have you heard of a Living Will before?

   [ ] Yes

> If YES is answered, from where or whom did you first learn of Living Wills?
>
> _____
> _____
> _____
> _____

   [ ] No

9. Do you have a good idea what a Living Will is?

   [ ] Yes

If YES is answered, please describe a Living Will _____

_____

Where did you get this understanding? _____

_____

_____

[ ] No

10. Have you heard of a Durable Power of Attorney for Health Care before?

[ ] Yes

If YES is answered, from where or whom did you first learn of a
Durable Power of Attorney for Health Care? _____

_____

_____

[ ] No

11. Do you have a good idea what a Durable Power of Attorney for Health
Care is?

[ ] Yes

If YES is answered, please describe a Durable Power of Attorney
for Health Care _____

_____

Where did you get this understanding? _____

_____

_____

[ ] No

12. Have you heard of the Arizona statute on Surrogate Decision Makers?

[ ] Yes

> If YES is answered, from where or whom did you first learn of the Arizona statute on Surrogate Decision Makers? _____
>
> _____
>
> _____

[ ] No

13. Do you have a good idea what the Arizona statute on Surrogate Decision Makers is?

   [ ] Yes

> If YES is answered, please describe the Arizona statute on Surrogate Decision Makers _____
>
> _____
>
> _____
>
> Where did you get this understanding? _____
>
> _____
>
> _____

[ ] No

14. Do you presently have a signed Living Will?

   [ ] Yes

> If YES is answered, what prompted you to get a Living Will?
>
> _____
>
> _____
>
> _____

[ ] No

15. Do you presently have a signed Durable Power of Attorney for Health Care?

   [ ] Yes

If YES is answered, what prompted you to get a Durable Power of
of Attorney for Health Care? _____

_____

_____

[ ] No

16. Assuming that you do not know all that is important regarding Living Wills
and Durable Power of Attorney for Health Care, will you want to learn
more about them?

[ ] Yes
[ ] No

17. Assuming that you have an interest to learn more, please identify below
your preferences for learning about Living Wills and Durable Power of
Attorney for Health Care. Check the boxes adjacent to the information
sources to describe your impression as to how appropriate each of the
sources would be. Check **one** for every source.

My physician
[ ] Very appropriate   [ ] Appropriate   [ ] Inappropriate
[ ] Very inappropriate
My lawyer
[ ] Very appropriate   [ ] Appropriate   [ ] Inappropriate
[ ] Very inappropriate
My clergy
[ ] Very appropriate   [ ] Appropriate   [ ] Inappropriate
[ ] Very inappropriate
A family member
[ ] Very appropriate   [ ] Appropriate   [ ] Inappropriate
[ ] Very inappropriate
A community class
[ ] Very appropriate   [ ] Appropriate   [ ] Inappropriate
[ ] Very inappropriate
My Pulmonary Rehabilitation Program
[ ] Very appropriate   [ ] Appropriate   [ ] Inappropriate
[ ] Very inappropriate
Private reading
[ ] Very appropriate   [ ] Appropriate   [ ] Inappropriate
[ ] Very inappropriate

18. How should discussions with a patient's physician regarding issues of Living Wills and Durable Powers of Attorney for Health Care be initiated?

  [ ] Physicians should initiate the discussion of the topic and provide information if the patient is interested

  [ ] Physicians should wait until patients initiate the discussion before information is provided to the patient

19. How would you perceive discussions by your physician regarding Living Wills and Durable Power of Attorney for Health Care?

  [ ] Informative

  [ ] Informative and reassuring

  [ ] Anxiety provoking but worthwhile because these discussions would be informative

  [ ] Too anxiety provoking to discuss

20. Have you had discussions with your physician regarding Living Wills and Durable Power or Attorney for Health Care?

  [ ] Yes

> If YES is answered, who initiated the discussions? _____
> _____
> _____
> _____

  [ ] No

> By the nature of our shared human condition, all of us with and without underlying medical conditions are at risk for serious sudden illnesses. Occasionally, some patients with sudden illnesses require the initiation of advanced life support measures, such as placement of a breathing tube in the throat and treatment in the intensive care unit with a mechanical ventilator (breathing machine). Some patients with serious illnesses may experience a cardiac arrest (heart stopping) and require cardiopulmonary resuscitation (pushing on the chest, placing an airway tube, applying electricity to the chest in an attempt to restart the heart beating). The following questions pertain to these issues.

21. Have you thought about the possibility that some day you might require placement of a breathing tube?

[ ] Yes

If YES is answered, do you have opinions whether you would approve of such treatment for yourself? _____

_____

_____

_____

[ ] No

22. Have you thought about the possibility that some day you might require treatment on a mechanical ventilator (breathing machine)?

[ ] Yes

If YES is answered, do you have opinions whether you would approve of such treatment for yourself? _____

_____

_____

_____

[ ] No

23. Have you thought about the possibility that some day you might require treatment with cardiopulmonary resuscitation (pushing on the chest, placing an airway tube, applying electricity to the chest in an attempt to restart the heart beating)?

[ ] Yes

If YES is answered, do you have opinions whether you would approve of such treatment for yourself? _____

_____

_____

_____

[ ] No

24. Would you want to discuss any thoughts regarding breathing tubes, mechanical ventilators, or cardiopulmonary resuscitation with any one?

[ ] Yes
[ ] No

25. Assuming that you would like to discuss these thoughts, please identify below your preferences for selecting persons for these discussions. Check the boxes adjacent to the persons that best describe how appropriate you believe they would be as participants in these discussions. Check **one** box for every person.

My physician
[ ] Very appropriate   [ ] Appropriate   [ ] Inappropriate
[ ] Very inappropriate
My lawyer
[ ] Very appropriate   [ ] Appropriate   [ ] Inappropriate
[ ] Very inappropriate
My clergy
[ ] Very appropriate   [ ] Appropriate   [ ] Inappropriate
[ ] Very inappropriate
A family member
[ ] Very appropriate   [ ] Appropriate   [ ] Inappropriate
[ ] Very inappropriate
A community class
[ ] Very appropriate   [ ] Appropriate   [ ] Inappropriate
[ ] Very inappropriate
My Pulmonary Rehabilitation Program
[ ] Very appropriate   [ ] Appropriate   [ ] Inappropriate
[ ] Very inappropriate

26. Assuming that you are under the regular care of a physician, when should discussions with your physician regarding issues of breathing tubes, mechanical ventilators, and cardiopulmonary resuscitation first be initiated? Select one of the responses.

[ ] When you are seen during routine office visits
[ ] When you are seen in the office with new serious illnesses
[ ] When you are admitted to the hospital for any reason
[ ] When you are admitted to the hospital with serious life-threatening illnesses
[ ] When you are hospitalized and have a serious illness that appears likely to require breathing tubes, mechanical ventilation, or cardiopulmonary resuscitation

27. How should discussions with a patient's physician regarding issues of breathing tubes, mechanical ventilators, and cardiopulmonary resuscitation be initiated?

    [ ] Physicians should initiate the discussion of the topic and provide information if the patient is interested.
    [ ] Physicians should wait until patients initiate the discussion before information is provided to the patient.

28. How would you perceive discussions by your physician regarding issues of breathing tubes, mechanical ventilators, and cardiopulmonary resuscitation?

    [ ] Informative
    [ ] Informative and reassuring
    [ ] Anxiety provoking but worthwhile because these discussions would be informative
    [ ] Too anxiety provoking to discuss

29. Have you had discussions with your physician regarding issues of breathing tubes, mechanical ventilators, and cardiopulmonary resuscitation?

    [ ] Yes

    ┌───┐
    │ If YES is answered, who initiated the discussions?_____ │
    │ _____   │
    │ _____   │
    └───┘

    [ ] No

30. Does an understanding exist between you and your physician whether you would accept or refuse treatment with either breathing tubes, mechanical ventilators, or cardiopulmonary resuscitation?

    [ ] We have discussed these issues, and an understanding exists
    [ ] We have discussed these issues, and we are developing an understanding of these issues
    [ ] We have not yet discussed these issues

31. Do you need any help in doing any of the following?

	Yes	No
shopping	[ ]	[ ]
walking	[ ]	[ ]
washing or bathing	[ ]	[ ]
eating	[ ]	[ ]
Have you been a patient in the ICU?	[ ]	[ ]

We want you to imagine how you would feel about your treatment if you were to develop a life threatening illness so severe that you would be very unlikely to survive without mechanical ventilation on an intensive care unit. We particularly want to know what factors or circumstances, such as the chances of recovery and your quality of life, would influence your decision to accept or refuse treatment.

Please read the following three questions and check the box opposite the statement with which you most agree.

32. Select **one** of the responses

   [ ] I would want mechanical ventilation started whatever the circumstances. Go to question 36.
   [ ] I would not want mechanical ventilation started whatever the circumstances. Go to question 36.
   [ ] I would want mechanical ventilation started only under certain circumstances. Proceed to question 33.

33. BEFORE this imaginary illness occurred, would you have wanted mechanical ventilation started if your health had deteriorated to the extent that you were

	YES	NO
Unable to walk well enough to get out of the house	[ ]	[ ]
Unable to walk without assistance	[ ]	[ ]
Unable to feed yourself without assistance	[ ]	[ ]
In constant pain	[ ]	[ ]
More forgetful but able to do most things	[ ]	[ ]
Unable to do favorite hobbies due to poor memory or concentration	[ ]	[ ]

34. Would you want mechanical ventilation started if your chances of a recovery were:

	YES	NO
Very good (better than a 9 out of 10 chance of recovery	[ ]	[ ]
Quite reasonable (approximately 7 or 8 out of 10 chance)	[ ]	[ ]
Fair (50:50 chance)	[ ]	[ ]
Poor (approximately 2 or 3 out of 10 chance)	[ ]	[ ]
Very poor (less than 1 in 10 chance of recovery)	[ ]	[ ]

35. Would you want mechanical ventilation started if following recovery you were:

	YES	NO
Left feeling as well as you presently do	[ ]	[ ]
Left feeling more tired all the time than you presently do	[ ]	[ ]
Left feeling more breathless than you presently do	[ ]	[ ]
Left in constant pain	[ ]	[ ]
Unable to do your favorite hobbies	[ ]	[ ]
Unable to walk well enough to get out of the house	[ ]	[ ]
Unable to walk without assistance	[ ]	[ ]
Unable to eat without assistance	[ ]	[ ]
More forgetful than usual, but still able to do most things	[ ]	[ ]
Too confused to be safely left alone	[ ]	[ ]

36. If you developed a severe illness that definitely required mechanical ventilation and you remained alert, who should make the decision whether you
should be treated with mechanical ventilation? Select **one** of the following choices.

[ ] I think that the medical and nursing staff should make the decision
about mechanical ventilation for me and I would rather not know too
many details about it

[ ] I think that the medical and nursing staff should make the decision
about mechanical ventilation for me, but only after explanation of
what it involves and the likely outcome

[ ] I think that the medical and nursing staff should explain what it
involves and the likely outcome, but leave the final decision to me

[ ] I think that the medical and nursing staff should explain what it
involves and the likely outcome to my family, and leave the final
decision to my family leaving me out of the discussion

37. If you were too ill to make a decision, who do you think should help
the medical and nursing staff to decide whether or not to commence
mechanical ventilation? Select **one** of the following choices.

[ ] No one. Leave it to the medical and nursing team.

[ ] Your relatives

[ ] Yourself in the form of a Living Will

[ ] A person formally selected by you in advance

38. Have you previously been hospitalized for your lung condition?

[ ] Yes

> If yes is answered, how many times have you been hospitalized for your lung condition?_____

[ ] No

39. Have you had previous intubations and episodes of mechanical ventilation due to your lung condition?
    [ ] Yes

> If yes is answered, how many previous intubations and episodes of mechanical ventilation have you experienced due to your lung condition?_____

[ ] No

40. Have you had previous episodes of mechanical ventilation for other conditions such as surgery?
    [ ] Yes

> If yes is answered, how many previous episodes of mechanical ventilation have you experienced for conditions other than your lung disease?
> _____
>
> Please describe the reason you received mechanical ventilation
> _____

[ ] No

From "Outcomes of advance directive education of pulmonary rehabilitation patients," by J. E. Heffner, B. Fahy, L. Hilling, and C. Barbieri, 1997, in *American Journal of Respiratory and Critical Care Medicine, 155,* pp. 1055-1059. Reprinted with permission.

END-OF-LIFE CARE DECISIONS QUESTIONNAIRE (EOLCDQII)

*Developed by Mary L. Stoeckle, Jane E. Doorley,
and Rosanna M. McArdle*

INSTRUMENT DEVELOPMENT, ADMINISTRATION, AND SCORING

Evaluating how well health professionals are implementing and complying with the Patient Self-Determination Act (PSDA) of 1990 is essential to improve practice and to determine why the policy initiative is or is not working. The EOLCDQII was developed to evaluate current beliefs and practices of physicians, nurses, pastoral care associates, and medical social workers regarding end-of-life care decisions. The instrument consists of a demographic section and two subscales of 10 questions each: perceptions scale (items 32, 33, 35, 36, 37, 40, 42, 44, 47, 48), and beliefs and practices scale (items 29, 30, 31, 34, 38, 39, 41, 43, 45, 46) (Stoeckle, Doorley, & McArdle, 1998).

PSYCHOMETRIC PROPERTIES

Content validity was assessed by a panel of experts including an intensivist physician with expertise in ethics, two doctorally prepared nurse researchers/ethicists, a director of pastoral care, and two critical care clinical nurse specialists. All items received 100% agreement by the experts for clarity and appropriateness. The instrument was administered to 409 health professionals. Cronbach's alpha was .85 for the perceptions of end-of-life process subscale, .73 for the beliefs and practices subscale, and .84 for the total scale. The subscales were established by factor analysis (Stoeckle et al., 1998).

SUMMARY AND CRITIQUE

The instrument is in early stages of psychometric development. It addresses the important function of compliance with the PSDA and developing professional, patient, and family education to support the law. To date, testing of the instrument has shown providers to be unsure about when an advance directive (AD) is needed and feeling that their work experience and educational preparation did not enable them to discuss end-of-life decisions with patients and families. Approximately one third believed that patients and families do not understand the information they are given about end-of-life decisions (Stoeckle et al., 1998).

Responses to selected items may be found in Stoeckle et al. (1998) and they recognize the limitations of a single site and convenience sample and recommend further testing of the instrument.

REFERENCE

Stoeckle, M. L., Doorley, J. E., & McArdle, R. M. (1998). Identifying compliance with end-of-life care decision protocols. *Dimensions of Critical Care Nursing, 17*(6), 314-321.

Instrument 5.7

\# _____

RN, Pastoral Care, Social Worker Demographic

END OF LIFE CARE DECISIONS QUESTIONNAIRE II

"By completing this questionnaire, I indicate my consent to participate in this study. I understand confidentiality will be maintained."

1. Age:

   _____20-24   _____35-39   _____50-54   _____65 or older
   _____25-29   _____40-44   _____55-59
   _____30-34   _____45-49   _____60-64

2. Gender:

   _____Male   _____Female

3. Ethnicity:

   _____African American
   _____Asian
   _____Caucasian
   _____Hispanic
   _____Native American
   _____Other   Specify_____

4. Marital Status:

   _____Married
   _____Widowed
   _____Divorced
   _____Separated
   _____Single

5. Religious Affiliation:

   _____Atheist
   _____Catholic
   _____Jewish
   _____Protestant   Specify_____
   _____None
   _____Other   Specify_____

6. Profession:

_____Chaplain/Pastoral Care   _____Full Time
_____Registered Nurse   _____Part Time
_____Social Worker

7. Highest level of education completed:

_____Diploma   _____Masters
_____Associate   _____Doctorate
_____Bachelors

8. What is your area of specialty?

_____Intensive Care Unit
_____Coronary Intensive Care Unit
_____Advanced Care Unit
_____Telemetry
_____Bone Marrow Transplant Unit
_____Burn Unit
_____Neuro Unit

9. Years of experience in specialty:

_____Less than 1 year   _____11-15 years
_____1-5 years   _____16-20 years
_____6-10 years   _____Greater than 20 years

10. Have you ever attended a course, seminar, or workshop on the Patient Self Determination Act?

_____Yes   _____No (If no, skip #11)

11. If yes, was this mandatory to fulfill a degree, work, or continuing education requirement?

_____Yes   _____No

12. Have you ever attended a course, seminar, or workshop concerning values, ethical, or moral development?

_____Yes   _____No (If no, skip #13)

13. If yes, was this mandatory to fulfill a degree, work, or continuing education requirement?

_____Yes   _____No

14. Have you, a family member, or a close friend ever had a life threatening experience or terminal illness?

    _____Yes   _____No

15. Has this life threatening experience or experience with terminal illness changed your beliefs, values, or attitude about death and dying?

    _____Yes   _____No

16. Has your personal experience with a life threatening event or terminal illness changed the way you approach end of life care discussions with patients and families?

    _____Yes   _____No

17. Have you discussed your end of life care wishes with your family?

    _____Yes   _____No

18. Have you completed advanced directives for yourself?

    _____Yes   _____No

19. Do you know your family's end of life care wishes?

    _____Yes   _____No

20. Have any of your family members completed advanced directives?

    _____Yes   _____No

21. A living will is a document that identifies what medical treatment you choose to omit or refuse in the event that you are unable to make those decisions for yourself AND are terminally ill.

    _____Agree   _____Disagree   _____Unsure

22. The definition of a durable power of attorney for healthcare is: appointment of a proxy to make medical decisions on your behalf when you can no longer decide for yourself.

    _____Agree   _____Disagree   _____Unsure

23. A durable power of attorney for healthcare applies when any illness or injury leaves you mentally incapacitated.

    _____Agree   _____Disagree   _____Unsure

24. There is no ethical difference between withholding life support measures or withdrawing these measures once started.

    _____Agree   _____Disagree   _____Unsure

25. Have you ever *initiated* a discussion about end of life decisions with patients or patients' families?

    _____Yes   _____No

    If yes, how many times have you *initiated* these discussions:

    _____less than 10 _____30-39 _____60-69 _____90-99
    _____10-19   _____40-49 _____70-79 _____100 or greater
    _____20-29   _____50-59 _____80-89 _____With ALL patients

26. How comfortable do you feel *initiating* end of life discussions with your patients?

    _____Very comfortable
    _____Somewhat comfortable
    _____Not comfortable at all

27. Do you think that additional education would enhance your ability to communicate with patients and families about end of life care?

    _____Agree   _____Disagree   _____Unsure

28. Who do you think should *initiate* discussions on end of life decisions? Please rank the following person(s) from 1 = highest priority to 8 = lowest priority, use 0 = NA (use each number only once).

    _____Chaplain/Pastoral Care Associate   _____Patient's Family
    _____Registered Nurse   _____Physician
    _____Pastor/Priest/Rabbi   _____Social Worker
    _____Patient   _____Other   Specify_____

_____

Physician Demographic

END OF LIFE CARE DECISIONS QUESTIONNAIRE II

"By completing this questionnaire, I indicate my consent to participate in this study. I understand confidentiality will be maintained."

1. Age:

    _____20-24   _____35-39   _____50-54   _____65 or older
    _____25-29   _____40-44   _____55-59
    _____30-34   _____45-49   _____60-64

2. Gender:

    _____Male   _____Female

3. Ethnicity:

    _____African American
    _____Asian
    _____Caucasian
    _____Hispanic
    _____Native American
    _____Other   Specify_____

4. Marital Status:

    _____Married
    _____Widowed
    _____Divorced
    _____Separated
    _____Single

5. Religious Affiliation:

    _____Atheist
    _____Catholic
    _____Jewish
    _____Protestant   Specify_____
    _____None
    _____Other   Specify_____

6. Profession:

_____Physician   _____Full time
_____Resident Physician   _____Part time

7. Highest level of education completed:

_____PhD
_____MD
_____DO

8. What is your area of specialty?

_____ Pulmonary/Thoracic
_____ Oncology
_____ Internal Medicine
_____ Surgery   Specify_____
_____ Neurology
_____ Nephrology
_____ Family Practitioner
_____ Other   Specify_____

9. Years of experience in specialty:

_____ Less than 1 year   _____ 11-15 years
_____ 1-5 years   _____ 16-20 years
_____ 6-10 years   _____ Greater than 20 years

10. Have you ever attended a course, seminar, or workshop on the Patient Self Determination Act?

_____ Yes   _____ No (If no, skip #11)

11. If yes, was this mandatory to fulfill a degree, work, or continuing education requirement?

_____ Yes   _____ No

12. Have you ever attended a course, seminar, or workshop concerning values, ethical or moral development?

_____ Yes   _____ No (If no, skip #13)

13. If yes, was this mandatory to fulfill a degree, work, or continuing education requirement?

_____ Yes   _____ No

14. Have you, a family member, or a close friend ever had a life threatening experience or terminal illness?

_____ Yes   _____ No

15. Has this life threatening experience or experience with terminal illness changed your beliefs, values, or attitude about death and dying?

_____ Yes   _____ No

16. Has your personal experience with a life threatening event or terminal illness changed the way you approach end of life care discussions with patients and families?

_____ Yes   _____ No

17. Have you discussed your end of life care wishes with your family?

_____ Yes   _____ No

18. Have you completed advanced directives for yourself?

_____ Yes   _____ No

19. Do you know your family's end of life care wishes?

_____ Yes   _____ No

20. Have any of your family members completed advance directives?

_____ Yes   _____ No

21. A living will is a document that identifies what medical treatment you choose to omit or refuse in the event that you are unable to make those decisions for yourself AND are terminally ill.

_____ Agree   _____ Disagree   _____ Unsure

22. The definition of a durable power of attorney for healthcare is: appointment of a proxy to make medical decisions on your behalf when you can no longer decide for yourself.

_____ Agree   _____ Disagree   _____ Unsure

23. A durable power of attorney for healthcare applies when any illness or injury leaves you mentally incapacitated.

_____ Agree   _____ Disagree   _____ Unsure

24. There is no ethical difference between withholding life support measures or withdrawing these measures once started.

    _____ Agree _____ Disagree _____ Unsure

25. Have you ever *initiated* a discussion about end of life decisions with patients or patients' families?

    _____ Yes _____ No

    If yes, how many times have you *initiated* these discussions:

    _____ less than 10 _____ 30-39 _____ 60-69 _____ 90-99
    _____ 10-19 _____ 40-49 _____ 70-79 _____ 100 or greater
    _____ 20-29 _____ 50-59 _____ 80-89 _____ With ALL patients

26. How comfortable do you feel *initiating* end of life discussions with your patients?

    ___ Very comfortable
    ___ Somewhat comfortable
    ___ Not comfortable at all

27. Do you think that additional education would enhance your ability to communicate with patients and families about end of life care?

    _____ Agree _____ Disagree _____ Unsure

28. Who do you think should *initiate* discussions on end of life decisions? Please rank the following person(s) from 1 = highest priority to 8 = lowest priority, use 0 = NA (use each number only once).

    _____ Chaplain/Pastoral Care Associate
    _____ Patient's Family
    _____ Registered Nurse   _____ Physician
    _____ Pastor/Priest/Rabbi   _____ Social Worker
    _____ Patient   _____ Other   Specify _____

Please read each statement concerning End of Life Care Decisions. Take your time and think about what each statement says. Beside each statement is a scale which ranges from strongly agree (SA) to strongly disagree (SD). For each item we would like you to circle the letters that represent the extent to which you agree or disagree with each statement. Please make sure that you answer EVERY ITEM and that you circle ONLY ONE letter(s) per item. Thank you for taking the time to complete this questionnaire.

SA = Strongly Agree
A = Agree
U = Undecided
D = Disagree
SD = Strongly Disagree

29. I believe my work experience enables me to   SA   A   U   D   SD
    discuss end of life care with patients and families.

30. I believe my education enables me to discuss end   SA   A   U   D   SD
    of life care with patients and families.

31. I feel comfortable using the words die/death   SA   A   U   D   SD
    when discussing end of life care with my patients
    or families.

32. Health care professionals provide patients   SA   A   U   D   SD
    and families with adequate information about
    end of life care choices.

33. The patient's wishes and details of end of life   SA   A   U   D   SD
    care discussions are recorded in the physician
    progress notes.

34. End of life care discussions facilitate physician-   SA   A   U   D   SD
    family agreement on treatment choices.

35. Terminally ill patients have adequate pain control. SA   A   U   D   SD

36. The patient's wishes and details of end of life   SA   A   U   D   SD
    care discussions are recorded in the nursing
    notes.

37. Patients understand the information they are   SA   A   U   D   SD
    given about end of life care.

38. I frequently discuss pain control for my terminally SA   A   U   D   SD
    ill patients with nurses/physicians.

39. All patients, even if they are not terminally ill, have the right to make decisions regarding end of life care (life support) even if that decision may lead to death.

SA   A   U   D   SD

40. Patients and families are given consistent information about the consequences of their end of life care decisions.

SA   A   U   D   SD

41. I frequently discuss pain control with my terminally ill patients.

SA   A   U   D   SD

42. Terminally ill patients have adequate resources available for evaluating pain.

SA   A   U   D   SD

43. Patients and families are often given options for treatment that are futile and prolong the dying process.

SA   A   U   D   SD

44. Patients and families are given adequate time for the process of making end of life care decisions.

SA   A   U   D   SD

45. I wait for the patient or family to initiate end of life care discussions.

SA   A   U   D   SD

46. I frequently collaborate with other healthcare professionals to facilitate end of life care decisions.

SA   A   U   D   SD

47. I believe patients and families are approached about end of life care decisions in an atmosphere that is nonthreatening and conducive to processing difficult decisions.

SA   A   U   D   SD

48. Patients and families are regularly included in update discussions regarding their end of life care decisions.

SA   A   U   D   SD

THANK YOU

SOURCE: From "Identifying compliance with end-of-life care decision protocols," by M. L. Stoekle, J. E. Doorley, and R. M. McArdle, 1998, *Dimensions of Critical Care Nursing, 17*(6), pp. 314-321. Copyright 1995. Permission for use must be obtained in writing from M. L. Stoekle, Ph.D., R.N., 5917 Lawrence Road, Cincinnati, OH 45248. Reprinted with permission.

Withdrawal of Life Support

There is a growing number of life-prolonging technologies, most frequently used to improve the short-term survival of patients with life-threatening illness in intensive care units (ICUs). These technologies must be used indefinitely to maintain benefit but they also have a substantial negative effect on the patient's quality of life. Decisions to withhold or withdraw treatment are increasingly common and may be a source of caregiver discomfort because such actions appear to breach expectations or promises to patients and family. Although there is an established consensus that patients may forego unwanted life-sustaining treatments, providers are frequently a part of these decisions.

The instruments reviewed in this section focus on how providers make such decisions. The studies that used these instruments found considerable variability among ICU providers responding to the same patient scenarios, suggesting that provider personal values were major determinants in their decisions. This is viewed as problematic, requiring regular interdisciplinary forums to build consensus on these issues (Cook et al., 1995).

REFERENCE

Cook, D. J., Guyatt, G. H., Jaeschke, R., Reeve, J., Spanier, A., King, D., Molloy, D. W., Willan, A., & Streiner, D. L. (1995). Determinants in Canadian health care workers of the decision to withdraw life support from the critically ill. *Journal of the American Medical Association, 273*, 703-708.

WITHDRAWAL OF LIFE SUPPORT IN CRITICALLY ILL PATIENTS

Developed by Deborah J. Cook, Gordon H. Guyatt,
Roman Jaeschke, Joan Reeve, Allen Spanier, Derek King,
D. Willie Molloy, Andrew Willan, and David L. Streiner
for the Canadian Critical Care Trials Group

INSTRUMENT DEVELOPMENT, ADMINISTRATION, AND SCORING

Little is known about how health care workers in intensive care units (ICUs) currently make decisions to withdraw and withhold life support. During this process, they attempt to fulfill several basic but often conflicting ethical obligations: to maintain life and to relieve suffering and as hope of recovery fades, to help achieve a peaceful and dignified death. The Withdrawal of Life Support in Critically Ill Patients instrument has been used to describe self-reported decision factors of these workers and to inform the debate about standards of end-of-life care (Cook et al., 1995).

Nurse and physician versions of the instrument differ primarily in the section that collects respondent demographic data. The main body of the instrument collects data about importance of various patient factors in the respondent's decision about withdrawal of life support. There are 12 scenarios; two sample scenarios are shown in Instrument 6.1 (pp. 195, 197). Although the scenarios vary several factors, they are constant in portraying the patient as not able to help with the decision and in having no family or friend available with whom to consult. This was done to avoid confounding the attitudes of health care workers with patient and family preferences (Cook et al., 1995).

PSYCHOMETRIC PROPERTIES

Literature search and interviews with ICU attending physicians, residents, and nurses were used to generate a list of factors contributing to the decision to withdraw life support, thus supporting content validity of the instrument. Common factors were patient's age, premorbid cognitive function, likelihood of surviving current episode, and likelihood of long-term survival. Intensivists, nurses, and methodologists rated scenarios' discriminality, clarity, utility, and face and content validity. Reliability for the 17 determinants of the withdrawal of life support, rated 2 weeks apart, ranged from .68 to .96. Mean scores on these may be found in Cook et al. (1995).

SUMMARY AND CRITIQUE

The instrument purports to measure what health care workers state they would do in response to scenarios; their actual practices were not observed. In addition, the relationship of responses to scenarios of this sort with responses in real clinical situations is generally not known.

The most important factors in the decision to withdraw life support included likelihood of surviving the current episode, likelihood of long-term survival, premorbid cognitive function, and patient age. Variability in respondents' choice of level of care was extensive in each scenario, with more than 10% of respondents choosing the opposite extreme. This contrasts with small variability in the importance ratings respondents gave to potential determinants of withdrawal of life support when asked independent of patient scenarios. These findings indicate that factors idiosyncratic to the providers were major determinants of their responses to withdraw care. The city or province in which care was provided could have as great an impact on health care workers' choices as whether the patient was 45 or 75 years of age (Cook et al., 1995).

In summary, the instrument Withdrawal of Life Support in Critically Ill Patients creates a structure within which to explore decision factors that providers report they use. Some initial information about validity and reliability is available.

REFERENCE

Cook, D. J., Guyatt, G. H., Jaeschke, R., Reeve, J., Spanier, A., King, D., Molloy, D. W., Willan, A., & Streiner, D. L. (1995). Determinants in Canadian health care workers of the decision to withdraw life support from the critically ill. *Journal of the American Medical Association, 273,* 703-708.

Instrument 6.1

Ratings of Determinants of the Withdrawal of Life Support*

Factor	Physician Score	Nurse Score
Likelihood of surviving current episode	6.3	6.1
Patient advance directives	6.3	6.3
Premorbid cognitive function†	5.9	5.5
Likelihood of long-term survival	5.6	5.6
Family directives	5.1	4.9
Premorbid physical function	5.0	5.2
Age‡	4.7	5.0
Risk of legal complications‡	3.9	4.8
Hospital policy‡	3.8	5.0
Compliance with medical care‡	3.2	4.4
Premorbid emotional function‡	2.6	3.8
Alcohol abuse‡	2.6	3.2
Drug abuse‡	2.4	3.1
Religious conviction‡	1.8	2.8
Ethnic background	1.6	1.8
Socioeconomic status	1.5	1.5
Religious affiliation‡	1.5	2.2

*Ratings are as follows: a rating of 7 indicates that a factor is extremely important; 5, moderately important; 3. minimally important; and 1, completely irrelevant.
†For difference between physicians and nurses, $p < .001$.
‡For difference between physicians and nurses, $p < .001$.

SOURCE: From "Determinants in Canadian health care workers of the decision to withdraw life support from the critically ill," by D. J. Cook, G. H. Guyatt, R. Jaeschke, J. Reeve, A. Spanier, D. King, D. W. Molloy, A. Willan, and D. L. Streiner, 1995, *Journal of the American Medical Association, 273*, pp. 703-708. Copyright 1995, American Medical Association. Reprinted with permission.

WITHDRAWAL OF LIFE SUPPORT IN CRITICALLY ILL PATIENTS—THE CANADIAN NATIONAL PERSPECTIVE

Thank you very much for donating your time to complete this questionnaire. We are administering this to both physicians and nurses in university-affiliated intensive care units across Canada, to learn about the current beliefs and attitudes toward maintaining life support in critically ill patients.

The goal of this questionnaire is to examine these attitudes, not to change or influence them. At no stage will we identify the respondents by name. All information obtained during this survey will be entirely confidential.

We thank you very much for your participation in this project.

Please record the time at which you start this questionnaire   [ ][ ] : [ ][ ]

Nurse Data Base

1. Your age (years) . . . . [ ]

2. Gender. . . . . [ ]
       1 = male
       2 = female

3. Year of diploma/degree . . . . [ ][ ][ ][ ]

4. Years of intensive care experience. . . . . [ ][ ]

5. Country of birth: _____

6. Country of nursing school graduation: _____

7. Religious affiliation . . . . [ ]
       1 = no religious affiliation
       2 = religious affiliation (please specify): _____

For Nurses:

1) In general, when you are considering the withdrawal of life support, how important are each of the following patient factors in making your decision? (Please circle appropriate response.)

    1   completely irrelevant
    2   unimportant
    3   minimally important
    4   somewhat important
    5   moderately important
    6   very important
    7   extremely important

age	1	2	3	4	5	6	7
premorbid cognitive function	1	2	3	4	5	6	7
compliance with medical care	1	2	3	4	5	6	7
ethnic background	1	2	3	4	5	6	7
premorbid emotional function	1	2	3	4	5	6	7
socioeconomic status/occupation	1	2	3	4	5	6	7
familial directives	1	2	3	4	5	6	7
patient advance directives	1	2	3	4	5	6	7
likelihood of surviving current episode	1	2	3	4	5	6	7
employment status	1	2	3	4	5	6	7
religious affiliation	1	2	3	4	5	6	7
religious conviction	1	2	3	4	5	6	7
drug abuse	1	2	3	4	5	6	7
likelihood of long term survival	1	2	3	4	5	6	7
alcohol abuse	1	2	3	4	5	6	7
risk of legal implications	1	2	3	4	5	6	7
hospital policy	1	2	3	4	5	6	7
premorbid physical function	1	2	3	4	5	6	7
others (please specify:_____)	1	2	3	4	5	6	7

2) ICU nurses may differ considerably in their ideas about and approaches to withdrawing life support. In thinking about you and your colleagues, where do you believe that you fit on this continuum? (Please circle the appropriate response.)

    In comparison to my colleagues' tendency to withdraw life support, I think I am

    1   much more likely
    2   more likely
    3   as likely

    4   less likely
    5   much less likely

Now we would like you to read the following two scenarios and answer the questions which follow, keeping in mind the patient described in each of the scenarios.

ICU Attending Data Base

1. Your age (years) . . . . [ ][ ]

2. Gender . . . . [ ]
       1 = male
       2 = female

3. Year of graduation from medical school . . . . [ ][ ][ ][ ]

4. Year of completion of post-graduate training . . . . [ ][ ][ ][ ]

5. In which program were you trained? (Please circle all that apply)
   Internal medicine 1
   respirology 2
   cardiology 3
   surgery 4
   anesthesia 5
   emergency medicine 6
   critical care medicine 7
   pediatrics 8
   other (please specify):_____ 9

6. Number of years you have been an ICU attending . . . . [ ][ ]

7. Percent of time spent in clinical work (In last year) . . . . [ ][ ][ ].[ ]

8. Percent of clinical time spent in ICU (in last year) . . . . [ ][ ][ ].[ ]

9. Country of birth: _____

10. Country of medical school graduation: _____

11. Religious affiliation . . . . [ ]
        1 = no religious affiliation
        2 = religious affiliation (please specify):_____

ICU Fellow/Resident/Intern Data Base

1. Your age (years) . . . . [ ][ ]

2. Gender . . . . [ ]
   1 = male
   2 = female
3. Year of graduation from medical school . . . . [ ][ ][ ][ ]

4. Months of Intensive care experience to date . . . . [ ][ ]

5. Year of completion of post-graduate training . . . . [ ][ ][ ][ ]

6. In which program were you currently enrolled? (Please circle all that apply)

   Internal medicine 1
   respirology 2
   cardiology 3
   surgery. 4
   anesthesia 5
   emergency medicine 6
   critical care medicine 7
   pediatrics 8
   other (please specify):_____ 9

7. Country of birth: _____

8. Country of medical school graduation: _____

9. Current status . . . . [ ]
   1 = Intern
   2 = resident
   3 = fellow

10. If resident specify year of training. . . . . [ ]

11. Religious affiliation. . . . . [ ]
   1 = no religious affiliation
   2 = religious affiliation (please specify):_____

ID Number: [ ][ ][ ][ ][ ][ ]

For Physicians:

1) In general, when you are considering the withdrawal of life support, how important are each of the following patient factors in making your decision? (Please circle appropriate response.)

    1   completely irrelevant
    2   unimportant
    3   minimally important
    4   somewhat important
    5   moderately important
    6   very important
    7   extremely important

	1	2	3	4	5	6	7
age	1	2	3	4	5	6	7
premorbid cognitive function	1	2	3	4	5	6	7
compliance with medical care	1	2	3	4	5	6	7
ethnic background	1	2	3	4	5	6	7
premorbid emotional function	1	2	3	4	5	6	7
socioeconomic status/occupation	1	2	3	4	5	6	7
familial directives	1	2	3	4	5	6	7
patient advance directives	1	2	3	4	5	6	7
likelihood of surviving current episode	1	2	3	4	5	6	7
employment status	1	2	3	4	5	6	7
religious affiliation	1	2	3	4	5	6	7
religious conviction	1	2	3	4	5	6	7
drug abuse	1	2	3	4	5	6	7
likelihood of long term survival	1	2	3	4	5	6	7
alcohol abuse	1	2	3	4	5	6	7
risk of legal implications	1	2	3	4	5	6	7
hospital policy	1	2	3	4	5	6	7
premorbid physical function	1	2	3	4	5	6	7
others (please specify:_____).	1	2	3	4	5	6	7

2) ICU physicians may differ considerably in their approach to withdrawing life support. In thinking about you and your colleagues (other Intensivists), where do you believe that you fit on this continuum? (Please circle the appropriate response.)

    In comparison to my colleagues' tendency to withdraw life support, I think I am

        1   much more likely
        2   more likely
        3   as likely
        4   less likely
        5   much less likely

Now we would like you to read the following two scenarios and answer the questions which follow, keeping in mind the patient described in each scenario.

Scenario #4

A 75-year-old woman was admitted to the ICU with urosepsis 10 days ago. She now requires two inotropes to maintain a mean arterial pressure of 80 mm Hg, is ventilator dependent, comatose and in acute oliguric renal failure. Her APACHE score is 38, suggesting a 10% chance of survival.

Her past history includes long-standing depression, responsive to treatment. She has been walking with a cane due to a chronic deformity from polio.

She used to run the family manufacturing business, which involved supervision of ten people. Until just before admission, she continued to do the bookkeeping for the firm. She is single, and lives alone in her own home.

There are no known written or verbal advance directives. The patient has an older brother living in the United States, with whom she has not spoken for years, and whose current whereabouts are not known. There are no other living relatives. A few friends visit her in the ICU, but none want to be involved in decisions regarding her medical care.

For Office Use:
pair2 case1 +–+–
pair7 case2 +–+–

3) Of the following approaches to this patient's care, which do you think would most likely be *in the patient's best interest* at this time? (Please circle the appropriate response.)

    1   allow the patient to die in a humane fashion
    2   continue with aggressive therapy for 24-48 hours, and see how it goes, with a plan to stop when the situation looks hopeless, but carry on if it looks good
    3   continue with aggressive therapy

4) Which of the following courses of action describe what you feel represents care that is most likely to be *in the patient's best interest*? (Please circle the appropriate response.)

    1   continue with full aggressive management and plan for dialysis if necessary
    2   continue with current management, add inotropic therapy, change antibiotics etc. as needed, but do not start dialysis

3   continue with current management but add no new therapeutic intervention
4   discontinue inotropes and other maintenance therapy but continue mechanical ventilation and comfort measures
5   discontinue inotropes and mechanical ventilation but continue comfort measures

5) How confident are you that the course of action you have chosen for this patient's care would be the one *in the patient's best interest*? (Please circle the appropriate response.)

1   very confident
2   moderately confident
3   somewhat confident
4   minimally confident
5   not at all confident

6) Now, we would like you to consider not only what you feel would be in the patient's best interest, but in addition, *all other factors that you feel bear on the decision*. Considering all of these factors (i.e., peer opinion, hospital policy, medicolegal issues), please choose the one approach that comes closest to *what you would do* if you were faced with the case described in this scenario at this time. (Please circle the appropriate response.)

1   continue with full aggressive management and plan for dialysis if necessary
2   continue with current management, add inotropic therapy, change antibiotics etc. as needed, but do not start dialysis
3   continue with current management but add no new therapeutic intervention
4   discontinue inotropes and other maintenance therapy but continue mechanical ventilation and comfort measures
5   discontinue inotropes and mechanical ventilation but continue comfort measures

7) How confident are you that the approach to this patient's care that you have chosen accurately reflects what *you would actually do* when confronted with this situation in the ICU? (Please circle the appropriate response.)

1   very confident
2   moderately confident
3   somewhat confident
4   minimally confident
5   not at all confident

Scenario #11

A 45-year-old woman was admitted to the ICU ten days ago with urosepsis. She requires one inotrope to maintain a mean arterial pressure of 80 mm Hg, is starting to be weaned from mechanical ventilation but has acute non-oliguric renal failure. Her APACHE score is 24, suggesting a 50% chance of survival.

Her past history includes long-standing depression, responsive to treatment, and breast cancer diagnosed five years ago. Three months prior to admission, she was found to have recurrent local disease with vertebral metastases and is now receiving palliative hormonal therapy. Her cancer-related one-year mortality rate is 90%. She has been walking with a cane since a serious motor vehicle accident during her teenage years.

She used to run the family manufacturing business, which involved supervision of ten people. However, her premorbid cognitive function has been limited by herpes encephalitis which she contracted two years ago. She now lives in a chronic care facility because of an inability to look after herself; she is able to feed and dress herself and carry on a simple conversation.

The patient is single. There are no known written or verbal advance directives. She has an older brother living in the United States, with whom she has not spoken for years, and whose current whereabouts are not known. There are no other living relatives. A few friends visit her in the ICU, but none want to be involved in decisions regarding her medical care.

For Office Use:
pair7 case1 –+–+–
pair2 case2 –+–+–
pair10 case2 –+–+–

8) Of the following approaches to this patient's care, which do you think would most likely be *in the patient's best interest* at this time? (Please circle the appropriate response.)

    1   allow the patient to die in a humane fashion
    2   continue with aggressive therapy for 24-48 hours, and see how it goes, with a plan to stop when the situation looks hopeless, but carry on if it looks good
    3   continue with aggressive therapy

9) Which of the following courses of action describe what you feel represents care that is most likely to be *in the patient's best interest*? (Please circle the appropriate response.)

    1   continue with full aggressive management and plan for dialysis if necessary

    2   continue with current management, add inotropic therapy, change antibiotics etc. as needed, but do not start dialysis

    3   continue with current management but add no new therapeutic intervention

    4   discontinue inotropes and other maintenance therapy but continue mechanical ventilation and comfort measures

    5   discontinue inotropes and mechanical ventilation but continue comfort measures

10) How confident are you that the course of action you have chosen for this patient's care would be the one *in the patient's best interest*? (Please circle the appropriate response.)

    1   very confident

    2   moderately confident

    3   somewhat confident

    4   minimally confident

    5   not at all confident

11) Now, we would like to consider not only what you feel would be in the patient's best interest, but in addition, *all other factors that you feel bear on the decision*. Considering all of these factors (i.e., peer opinion, hospital policy, medicolegal issues), please choose the one approach that comes closest to *what you would do* if you were faced with the case described in this scenario at this time. (Please circle the appropriate response.)

    1   continue with full aggressive management and plan for dialysis if necessary

    2   continue with current management, add inotropic therapy, change antibiotics etc. as needed, but do not start dialysis

    3   continue with current management but add no new therapeutic intervention

    4   discontinue inotropes and other maintenance therapy but continue mechanical ventilation and comfort measures

    5   discontinue inotropes and mechanical ventilation but continue comfort measures

12) How confident are you that the approach to this patient's care that you have chosen accurately reflects what *you would actually do* when confronted with this situation in the ICU? (Please circle the appropriate response.)

  1   very confident
  2   moderately confident
  3   somewhat confident
  4   minimally confident
  5   not at all confident

13) Please record the time that you finished these forms   [ ][ ] : [ ][ ]

Thank you very much for your time.

WILLINGNESS TO WITHDRAW LIFE SUPPORT (WWLS)

Developed by Nicholas A. Christakis
and David A. Asch

INSTRUMENT DEVELOPMENT, ADMINISTRATION, AND SCORING GUIDELINES

Although the right of competent adults to make decisions to withdraw life support is well established, the manner by which critically ill patients should die is usually entrusted to physicians. These patients may be on several types of life support at once, any of which might be withdrawn, and the decision about which to withdraw at what time may influence the rapidity, painlessness, and dignity of patients' deaths (Christakis & Asch, 1993).

The WWLS solicits both physicians' self-reported preferences and responses to experimentally varied clinical vignettes. In addition to a fixed set of direct questions about respondents' preferences (e.g., see Figure 1 in Instrument 6.2), decision-oriented questions accompany seven clinical vignettes. Some deal with iatrogenic complications (see Figure 3 in Instrument 6.2, which replaces the last sentence of the first paragraph in the control vignette).

In all of the vignettes, the patient is terminally ill and comatose, has clearly expressed in advance a desire for life support to be withdrawn under these circumstances, and the family has agreed with that decision. Thus, the decision to withdraw life support has already been made. The withdrawal of life support should be least controversial for such patients and be least subject to potential biases. Respondents indicate their likelihood of withdrawing particular life support by a 1 (low willingness) to a 5 (high willingness). Mean response was 3.5 (Christakis & Asch, 1995).

PSYCHOMETRIC PROPERTIES

The WWLS was reviewed by two experts in critical care and pre-tested with ten internists. It was then administered to 485 physicians at one university medical center. Cronbach's alpha was .79, and factor analysis supported one underlying factor. There was considerable variability in internists' willingness to withdraw life-sustaining therapy. An attitude of greater willingness was associated with a higher self-reported frequency of having done so, supportive of validity (Christakis & Asch, 1995).

SUMMARY AND CRITIQUE

Description of means by which content validity was established, including the rationale for choice of technologies, did not seem clear. Christakis and Asch note that responses to scenarios may not reflect behavior in real clinical situations, in which matters are discussed with family and colleagues and when more than one form of life support may be withdrawn at the same time. Self-reports of frequency of withdrawal may be unreliable (Christakis & Asch, 1993).

Use of the instrument showed that the physicians studied preferred to withdraw forms of therapy supporting organs that failed for natural rather than iatrogenic reasons, to withdraw recently instituted rather than long-standing interventions, to withdraw forms of therapy resulting in immediate death, and to withdraw forms of therapy resulting in delayed death when confronted with diagnostic uncertainty (Christakis & Asch, 1993).

Christakis and Asch's concern is that in following these "biases," physicians may not be supporting patients' humanity by prolonging the period of dying, increasing suffering of patients and families, wasting resources, and raising concerns about patient goals and autonomy. When formulating ADs, patients tend not to make distinctions among various forms of life support, but some physicians apparently do. That nearly half of the respondents were either neutral or unwilling to withdraw life support in these uncontroversial situations is congruent with other studies that show that physicians are devoted to life-sustaining technology once it is implemented.

This can occur even though patients and family have made the decision to withdraw (Christakis & Asch, 1993).

The WWLS might be used to document biases of the physicians involved and to provoke consideration of how these might be communicated to involved patients, in the spirit of full disclosure (Christakis & Asch, 1993). Further work on validity should be accomplished.

REFERENCES

Christakis, N. A., & Asch, D. A. (1993). Biases in how physicians choose to withdraw life support. *The Lancet, 342,* 642-646.
Christakis, N. A., & Asch, D. A. (1995). Physician characteristics associated with decisions to withdraw life support. *American Journal of Public Health, 85,* 367-372.

Instrument 6.2

WILLINGNESS TO WITHDRAW LIFE SUPPORT (WWLS)

Some physicians may feel differently about withdrawing life-sustaining therapy depending upon whether that therapy supports an organ system that has failed for natural or for iatrogenic reasons. All else being equal, which of the following medical therapies would you prefer to withdraw? 1) a treatment that the patient has required because of his underlying disease; or 2) a treatment that the patient has required because of an iatrogenic complication.

Figure 1: Example of direct question

SL is a 68-year-old patient of yours with no significant past medical history. Eight days ago she suffered a prolonged seizure complicated by hypotension, myoglobinuria, acute renal failure, and severe obtudation. She now requires hemodialysis. A chest x-ray on admission showed a mass in the right mid-lung field. A CT scan of the brain showed multiple brain metastases. You decided a diagnostic bronchoscopy was needed and you consulted a pulmonologist to perform it. Bronchoscopic biopsy of the mass showed squamous cell carcinoma. Her later course was complicated by a massive pulmonary haemorrhage, and she has required mechanical ventilation in addition to hemodialysis. The patient has required mechanical ventilation and daily dialysis for one week, and her mental status has not improved. SL had previously expressed the wish to her family and to you that should she suffer a medical catastrophe, she would prefer to die rather than be kept alive by artificial means. Because of these previously expressed wishes, her family asks that you withdraw life support.

Figure 2: Control vignette

Unfortunately, through an error in technique, the bronchoscopy was performed with the wrong type of biopsy needle, resulting in a massive pulmonary haemorrhage. Because of this iatrogenic complication, she has required mechanical ventilation in addition to hemodialysis.

Figure 3: Vignette with iatrogenic complication

SOURCE: From "Biases in how physicians choose to withdraw life support," by N. A. Christakis and D. A. Asch, 1993, *The Lancet, 342,* pp. 642-646. Reprinted with permission.

NOTE: To obtain a copy of the WWLS and for permission to use it, contact Dr. Christakis at the University of Chicago Medical Center.

Aggressiveness of Care

Decision making about the level of aggressiveness of treatment, from comfort care to full therapeutic endeavor, is believed to be central to quality of care. Such a decision is basically about value of the treatment, its good and harm to the patient and to the community. Choices include the utilitarian prediction of outcome, the relational ethic of caring, or a combination of principle-based ethics with caring. Decision making for the level of aggressiveness also is an important part of the quality of care for patients. Frequently, there is no single correct decision (Baggs, 1993).

Provider disagreement about the appropriate level of aggressiveness is not uncommon and often reflects different values by discipline (Baggs & Schmitt, 1995). Frequently, nurses support patient autonomy more strongly than do physicians, who believe they alone should make life-and-death decisions for unconscious patients in the intensive care unit (ICU). The instruments in this section focus on settings (ICUs) and situations (do not resuscitate) in which these disagreements are most common. Because they describe the basis on which such decisions are made, the instruments can be used to negotiate an appropriate level of aggressiveness.

REFERENCES

Baggs, J. G. (1993). Collaborative interdisciplinary bioethical decision making in intensive care units. *Nursing Outlook, 41*(3), 108-111.

Baggs, J. G., & Schmitt, M. H. (1995). Intensive care decisions about level of aggressiveness of care. *Research in Nursing and Health 18,* 345-355.

DECISIONS ABOUT AGGRESSIVENESS OF CARE (DAC) DECISIONS ABOUT AGGRESSIVENESS OF CARE FOR SPECIFIC PATIENTS (DAC[SP])

Developed by Judith Gedney Baggs
and Madeline H. Schmitt

INSTRUMENT DEVELOPMENT, ADMINISTRATION, AND SCORING

One important set of ethical decisions in intensive care settings concerns choosing how aggressively to treat patients, from comfort care to full therapeutic endeavor. Such decisions are an important part of care for the critically ill but are complex because there is no single correct decision. Earlier studies have demonstrated differences in the level of care that nurses and physicians believe is appropriate and the poor communication between them about that decision making. Such differences can obstruct potential patient benefits and provider satisfaction that can flow from more collaborative decision making. These instruments were designed to measure providers' perceptions about choices related to level of aggressiveness of care (Decisions About Aggressiveness of Care or DAC) and those same perceptions in reference to a specific patient (Decisions About Aggressiveness of Care for Specific Patients or DAC[SP]). They have so far been used in research investigating involvement in level of care decisions and providers' satisfaction with that process (Baggs & Schmitt, 1995).

DAC[SP] should be administered to the nurse and physician caring for a particular patient at approximately the same time so that patient condition would be the same for both. Comparisons can then be made between responses from the two professionals (Baggs & Schmitt, 1995).

There is no overall score; groups are compared by their answers to individual questions. Questions 1 and 2 on the DAC were used to identify most important factors, with Question 1 determining frequency with which providers marked it, and with Question 2 determining what they identified as the most important factors. For Questions 3 through 6, between-group and within-group differences were compared, and the number of people who should be involved were compared with the total who actually were involved. Questions 7, 8, and 9 are scored as numbered. To date, no norms are available (J. G. Baggs, personal communication, 1998).

PSYCHOMETRIC PROPERTIES

The instruments incorporated evidence from the literature and were reviewed for content validity by nurse and physician experts in intensive care units. Experts were asked if questions and the instrument as a whole were relevant to and represented the construct of interdisciplinary bioethical decision making in ICUs. A pilot study showed that there was significant variance in response, which indicates that a full range of the variable was being examined and that responses differed between providers. Test-retest reliability of the DAC across a 2-week period was .73. No reliability estimate during this period is possible for the DAC[SP] because the patients' conditions cannot be expected to remain constant. Internal consistency reliability was .74 for the discussion and agreement questions on the DAC. In further work, 314 decisions were studied with DAC[SP] (Baggs & Schmitt, 1995).

Nurses and resident physicians agreed that the three most important factors influencing level of aggressiveness of care decisions were patient request, possibility of benefit, and diagnosis. More than 20% of the time both groups believed more care was being provided than was appropriate (Baggs & Schmitt, 1995).

SUMMARY AND CRITIQUE

The general purpose of these instruments is to study providers' perceptions of making ethical decisions about level of aggressiveness of care in ICUs. By comparing nurses and physicians, and comparing those general responses to ones related to specific patients and decisions made about their care, the two instruments provide the basis for measuring what providers believe generally happens. Baggs and Schmitt also indicate that these instruments may be modified to examine other types of decisions such as to withdraw or withhold care, to extubate patients, or to transfer or discharge patients (Baggs, 1993b).

The DAC and the DAC[SP] are in an early stage of development. Thus far data have been collected from residents and nurses in a teaching hospital. No reported evidence of construct validity could be located. Much of the information about how clinical ethical decisions are made in ICUs and who care providers believe should be involved suggests problems in nurse-physician decision making in the area of aggressiveness of care (Baggs, 1993a). Examination of these beliefs in a particular set of providers could presumably form the basis for mutual collaboration.

A significant body of research shows that interdisciplinary collaboration in intensive care and other settings is associated with better patient outcomes, controlling for severity of illness (Baggs, Ryan, Phelps, Richeson, & Johnson, 1992). That particular score patterns indicating collaborative decision making about level of aggressiveness of care as measured by the DAC and DAC[SP] yields better patient outcomes could not be verified.

REFERENCES

Baggs, J. G. (1993a). Collaborative interdisciplinary bioethical decision making in intensive care units. *Nursing Outlook, 41,* 108-111.

Baggs, J. G. (1993b). Two instruments to measure interdisciplinary bioethical decision making. *Heart and Lung, 22,* 542-547.

Baggs, J. G. (1998). Electronic message to author.

Baggs, J. G., Ryan, S. A., Phelps, C. E., Richeson, J. F., & Johnson, J. E. (1992). The association between interdisciplinary collaboration and patient outcomes in a medical intensive care unit. *Heart and Lung, 21,* 18-24.

Baggs, J. G., & Schmitt, M. H. (1995). Intensive care decisions about level of aggressiveness of care. *Research in Nursing and Health, 18,* 345-355.

Instrument 7.1

Code: _____

DECISIONS ABOUT
AGGRESSIVENESS OF CARE (DAC)

Please respond to all questions in terms of the usual practice on *this medical ICU*.

1. Mark the factors from the list below that influence your judgments when you are involved in decision making about aggressiveness of care (from comfort care to full therapeutic endeavor) for an ICU patient. Check all that apply.

    _____ 1. Age of patient
    _____ 2. Diagnosis (nature of underlying illness)
    _____ 3. Family's (significant other's) requests
    _____ 4. Financial impact of illness/care
    _____ 5. Lack of family (significant other)
    _____ 6. Limited ICU bed availability
    _____ 7. Patient discomfort from treatment
    _____ 8. Patient's functional status
    _____ 9. Patient's mental status
    _____ 10. Patient's requests (present or past)
    _____ 11. Probability of benefit from treatment/care
    _____ 12. Productivity (contribution to society) of patient
    _____ 13. Quality of life
    _____ 14. Other (write in)_____

2. What are the three most important factors influencing your judgments in decision making about aggressiveness of care (from most [1] to least [3] important)? You may write in numbers of items above or fill in the blanks.

    1._____
    2._____
    3._____

3. Who *should be* involved in making decisions about aggressiveness of treatment for MICU patients *capable of participating* in health care decisions? (Check all that apply)

    _____1. attending physician
    _____2. chaplain
    _____3. close family/significant other

____4. consulting physicians
____5. ethics consultant
____6. house officers
____7. nurses
____8. patient
____9. other _____

4. In this MICU who *actually is* involved in making decisions about aggressiveness of care for patients *capable of participating* in health care decisions?
   ____1. attending physician
   ____2. chaplain
   ____3. close family/significant other
   ____4. consulting physicians
   ____5. ethics consultant
   ____6. house officers
   ____7. nurses
   ____8. patient
   ____9. other_____

5. Who *should be* involved in making decisions about aggressiveness of
   treatment for MICU patients who are *NOT capable of participating* in
   health care decisions?
   ____1. attending physician
   ____2. chaplain
   ____3. close family/significant other
   ____4. consulting physicians
   ____5. ethics consultant
   ____6. house officers
   ____7. nurses
   ____8. patient (prior expression of wishes)
   ____9. other_____

6. In this MICU who *actually is* involved in making decisions about aggressiveness of care for patients who are *NOT capable of participating* in health
   care decisions?
   ____1. attending physician
   ____2. chaplain
   ____3. close family/significant other
   ____4. consulting physicians
   ____5. ethics consultant
   ____6. house officers
   ____7. nurses
   ____8. patient (prior expression of wishes)
   ____9. other_____

7. Generally, how satisfied are you with the way decisions about aggressiveness of care are made (the decision making process) in this MICU? (Circle response that best represents your judgment)

1	2	3	4	5	6	7
Not Satisfied						Fully Satisfied

8. Is there generally *discussion* in this MICU about decisions on aggressiveness of care for patients? (Please circle an answer for each question.)

	Rarely	Occaionally	Sometimes	Frequently	Almost Always
• Among physicians	1	2	3	4	5
• Among nurses	1	2	3	4	5
• Between nurses and physicians	1	2	3	4	5
• Between nurses and the patient	1	2	3	4	5
• Between physicians and the patient	1	2	3	4	5
• Between nurses and the family/significant other	1	2	3	4	5
• Between physicians and the family/significant other	1	2	3	4	5
• Between the patient and the family/significant other	1	2	3	4	5

9. Is there generally *agreement* in this MICU about decisions on aggressiveness of care for patients? (Please circle an answer for each question.)

	Rarely	Occaionally	Sometimes	Frequently	Almost Always
• Among physicians	1	2	3	4	5
• Among nurses	1	2	3	4	5
• Between nurses and physicians	1	2	3	4	5
• Between nurses and the patient	1	2	3	4	5
• Between physicians and the patient	1	2	3	4	5
• Between nurses and the family/significant other	1	2	3	4	5
• Between physicians and the family/significant other	1	2	3	4	5
• Between the patient and the family/significant other	1	2	3	4	5

6/9/92

SOURCE: Developed based on Baggs, 1990; Frampton & Mayewski, 1987; Smedira et al., 1990; Youngner, Jackson, & Allen, 1979. © J. Baggs, 1992. From "Two instruments to measure interdisciplinary bioethical decision making," by J. G. Baggs, 1993, *Heart & Lung, 22,* 542-547. Reprinted with permission.

Instrument 7.2

DECISIONS ABOUT AGGRESSIVENESS
OF CARE FOR SPECIFIC PATIENT DAC(SP)

These two pages to be completed by data collector.

1. Patient Code: _____   1a.   Attending MD Code: _____

2. Length of MICU stay (hours): _____ 3. Sex: _____

4. Age: _____

4a. Race: _____ American Indian or Alaskan Native

_____ Asian or Pacific Islander

_____ Black, not Hispanic

_____ Hispanic

_____ White, not Hispanic

5. Primary reason for ICU admission (diagnosis, system failure):

_____

6. Do the MD and RN agree that the nurse was involved in decision making? [DAC(SP) interview questions 4]

____ No
____ Yes

7. Do the MD and RN agree that the patient was involved in decision making? [DAC(SP) interview questions 4]

____ No
____ Yes

8. Do the MD and RN agree that family/significant other was involved in decision making? [DAC(SP) interview questions 4]

____ No
____ Yes

Resident Code: _____

9. From this resident's DAC question 3 (if MD believes pt is capable) or 5 (if resident believes pt is not capable). Should nurse be involved in decision making?

    ____ No
    ____ Yes

10. From this resident's DAC question 3 or 5. Should patient be involved?

    ____ No
    ____ Yes

11. From this resident's DAC question 3 or 5. Should family/significant other be involved?

    ____ No
    ____ Yes

12. This resident's CPS score _____

Nurse Code: _____

13. From this nurse's DAC question 3 (if nurse believes pt is capable) or 5 (if nurse believes pt is not capable). Should nurse be involved in decision making?

    ____ No
    ____ Yes

14. From this nurse's DAC question 3 or 5. Should patient be involved?

    ____ No
    ____ Yes

15. From this nurse's DAC question 3 or 5. Should family/significant other be involved?

    ____ No
    ____ Yes

16. This nurse's CPS score _____

Instrument 7.3

DAC(SP) CARE PROVIDER
INTERVIEW NURSE

Patient Code: _____ RN Code: _____

Please answer referring to the specific patient identified. Circle the best response.

1. Is the patient capable of participating in decision making about level of aggressiveness of her/his care?

YES   NO

2. How would you *characterize the level* of aggressiveness of care being provided for this patient?

1	2	3	4	5
DNR	DNR	Withhold	CPR, but	Full
Comfort	Maintain	only	with some	therapeutic
care	present	CPR	limitations	measures
only	treatments		on care	
	Do not add			
	new ones			

3. What do you *believe would be the appropriate level* of aggressiveness of care for this patient?

1	2	3	4	5
DNR	DNR	Withhold	CPR, but	Full
Comfort	Maintain	only	with some	therapeutic
care	present	CPR	limitations	measures
only	treatments		on care	
	Do not add			
	new ones			

4. Who was involved in making decisions about the level of aggressiveness of care for this patient? (Mark all that apply)

    _____ 1. attending physician
    _____ 2. chaplain
    _____ 3. close family/significant other
    _____ 4. consulting physicians

_____ 5. ethics consultant
_____ 6. house officers
_____ 7. nurses
_____ 8. patient
_____ 9. patient (prior expression of wishes)
_____ 10. other _____

5.   What were the three most important factors that influenced decision
     making about level of aggressiveness of care for this patient (from most
     to least important)? Write in numbers from list below or fill in blanks.

             1. _____

             2. _____

             3. _____

     1. Age of patient
     2. Diagnosis (nature of underlying illness)
     3. Family's (significant other's) requests
     4. Financial impact of illness/care
     5. Lack of family (significant other)
     6. Limited ICU bed availability
     7. Patient discomfort from treatment
     8. Patient's functional status
     9. Patient's mental status
     10. Patient's requests (present or past)
     11. Probability of benefit from treatment/care
     12. Productivity (contribution to society) of patient
     13. Quality of life

Instrument 7.4

DAC(SP) CARE PROVIDER
INTERVIEW RESIDENT

Patient Code: _____   MD Code: _____

Please answer referring to the specific patient identified. Circle the best response.

1. Is the patient capable of participating in decision making about level of aggressiveness of her/his care?

YES   NO

2. How would you *characterize the level* of aggressiveness of care being provided for this patient?

1	2	3	4	5
DNR	DNR	Withhold	CPR, but	Full
Comfort	Maintain	only	with some	therapeutic
care	present	CPR	limitations	measures
only	treatments		on care	
	Do not add			
	new ones			

3. What do you *believe would be the appropriate level* of aggressiveness of care for this patient?

1	2	3	4	5
DNR	DNR	Withhold	CPR, but	Full
Comfort	Maintain	only	with some	therapeutic
care	present	CPR	limitations	measures
only	treatments		on care	
	Do not add			
	new ones			

4. Who was involved in making decisions about the level of aggressiveness of care for this patient?

_____ 1. attending physician
_____ 2. chaplain
_____ 3. close family/significant other
_____ 4. consulting physicians

_____ 5. ethics consultant
_____ 6. house officers
_____ 7. nurses
_____ 8. patient
_____ 9. patient (prior expression of wishes)
_____10. other_____

5. What were the three most important factors that influenced decision making about level of aggressiveness of care for this patient (from most to least important)? Write in numbers from list below or fill in blanks.

1._____

2._____

3._____

1. Age of patient
2. Diagnosis (nature of underlying illness)
3. Family's (significant other's) requests
4. Financial impact of illness/care
5. Lack of family (significant other)
6. Limited ICU bed availability
7. Patient discomfort from treatment
8. Patient's functional status
9. Patient's mental status
10. Patient's requests (present or past)
11. Probability of benefit from treatment/care
12. Productivity (contribution to society) of patient
13. Quality of life

SOURCE: © J. Baggs, 1992. Reprinted with permission.

AGGRESSIVENESS OF NURSING CARE SCALE (ANCS)

Developed by Sonya Iverson Shelley, Rona Michele Zahorchak,
and Carol D. S. Gambrill

APPROPRIATENESS OF CARE QUESTIONNAIRE (ACQ)

Developed by David A. Sherman
and Kay Branum

BACKGROUND

Health professionals have disagreed about the type and level of intervention that should be provided a patient with a do-not-resuscitate (DNR) order. A process to identify areas of disagreement would be helpful for examining rationale for DNR care policy statements for the diverse needs of critically ill patients. Nurses frequently have specific concerns because they are deliverers of much of this care by virtue of their 24-hour-a-day responsibilities and because they have historically been excluded from DNR decision making.

Although patient classification schemes to guide access to elements and levels of care have been developed, a need remains for a standardized tool by which to study caregiver attitudes toward appropriate aggressiveness of care for these patients (Shelley, Zahorchak, & Gambrill, 1987).

INSTRUMENT DEVELOPMENT, ADMINISTRATION, AND SCORING

Shelley, Zahorchak, and Gambrill (1987) developed the Aggressiveness of Nursing Care Scale (ANCS) to measure attitudes toward aggressiveness of care. Aggressive physical care was defined as nursing actions aimed at curing the underlying illness and monitoring the patient's progress toward wellness and could include such measures as admission to the intensive care unit and beginning total parenteral nutrition. Comfort care, or nonaggressive physical care, was viewed as nursing actions directed at minimizing discomfort without specific or direct attention to the underlying disease and condition; these efforts include food or fluids as tolerated but without the use of tubes, minimal suctioning, and turning only within a patient's pain tolerance, dictated by the patient's disease and comfort.

The ANCS used a vignette (see Instrument 7.5) that varied the age of the patient (32-years-old or 72-years-old) and by inclusion or not of DNR orders, with participants then indicating with answers to 13 items how they would care for this patient on a 6-point Likert scale (1 = strongly agree to 6 = strongly disagree). Scores could range from 13 (for agreement with nonaggressive care) to 78 (representing agreement with extremely aggressive care). Scores lower than 35 reflect intent to provide minimum yet ethically defensible care, scores of 35 to 56 designate agreement with moderately aggressive care, and scores greater than 56 represent very aggressive care directed toward cure. Scores among ICU staff nurses and nursing students ranged from 19 to 75 with a mean of 52.8 and standard deviation of 10.8.

Forrester (1990) developed six vignettes by varying AIDS-related risk factors (gay vs. intravenous drug users), medical diagnosis (AIDS vs. non-AIDS), and DNR orders (DNR order vs. no DNR order) (see Instrument 7.5a) and used the same 13-item questionnaire as did Shelley et al. (1987) to measure nurses' attitudes toward aggressiveness of care. The 600 registered nurses employed in the mid-Atlantic region who volunteered to complete this version of the ANCS showed that AIDS-related risk factors did not influence ANCS scores. A non-AIDS diagnosis and DNR orders significantly decreased aggressiveness of nursing care attitudes, again in the moderately aggressive range.

Sherman and Branum (1995) have developed yet another version of the ANCS for critical care settings (Appropriateness of Care Questionnaire or ACQ). The vignette describing a patient with severe sepsis varied not only by DNR versus no DNR but also included psychosocial care items. Mean scores were 60.7 for the DNR group and 69.6 for the non-DNR group, with the groups differing only on the physical subscale. All items in the original questionnaire (Shelley et al., 1987) were retained, and six items were added to investigate emotional support of patients. Each was considered a subscale with a 20th item added about allocation of the nurse's resources outside the subscales. A 6-point numeric scale was used, anchored at each end from strongly agree (1) to strongly disagree (6).

The ACQ was pilot tested with five nurses; the average amount of time to complete it was 7 minutes. Scores are sums of individual items. The ACQ was tested with 87 nurses working in ICUs.

PSYCHOMETRIC PROPERTIES

For the ANCS, 30 routine nursing care actions that might vary depending on whether DNR orders were written for a patient were generated by a panel of four experienced nurses, supplemented and rewritten based on literature review. In the interest of greater comfort, it was believed that the care described in each item could ethically be withheld for a patient with a DNR. Content validity was judged by 25 experienced staff nurses. Study of internal consistency showed a Cronbach's alpha of .81 (Shelley et al., 1987). Forrester's version of the scale showed a coefficient alpha of .80 (Forrester, 1990). The ACQ showed a Cronbach's alpha of .84 for the physical subscale and .79 for the psychosocial subscale (scales confirmed by factor analysis) (Sherman & Branum, 1995).

SUMMARY AND CRITIQUE

Shelley et al. (1987) found that both greater age and DNR orders reduced aggressiveness of nursing care attitudes and that although attitudes were generally in the moderate range, nurses did not agree on what constituted comfort care.

A major limitation of the technique of simulation measurement is the possible discrepancy with actual behaviors in real clinical settings. In addition, focusing on the level of care for one specific patient limits generalizability to other critically ill patients. As originally developed, the ANCS focused only on physical care largely under control of nurses and did not include medications or emotional support to the patient and family. Both of these excluded areas are important to the care of patients in the situations depicted. It is expected that today these areas of care would yield different response patterns (Shelley et al., 1987).

No studies of validity other than content validity could be located. Changes in practice conditions in the 14 years since the ANCS was developed could affect a current assessment of content validity.

The ACQ does not include care issues such as pain control and some monitoring. The vignettes do not specify religion.

REFERENCES

Forrester, D. A. (1990). AIDS-related risk factors, medical diagnoses, do-not-resuscitate orders and aggressiveness of nursing care. *Nursing Research, 39*, 350-354.

Shelley, S. I., Zahorchak, R. M., & Gambrill, C. D. S. (1987). Aggressiveness of nursing care for older patients and those with do-not-resuscitate orders. *Nursing Research, 36*, 157-162.

Sherman, D. A., & Branum, K. (1995). Critical care nurses' perceptions of appropriate care of the patient with orders not to resuscitate. *Heart and Lung, 24*, 321-329.

Instrument 7.5a

Francis is a 72-year-old patient with fulminating resistant-pseudomonas sepsis in your unit. After 3 weeks of aggressive antibiotic therapy, there has been no clinical improvement. Francis is lethargic, but easily aroused. Due to the poor prognosis of this case and at the request of the patient and immediate family members, a Do-Not-Resuscitate order has been written.

The last sentence was deleted on the vignette questionnaires depicting the patient without DNR orders.

In some versions, the patient's age was 28 years.

Aggressiveness of Care Scale

ITEMS	Strongly agree					Strongly disagree
1. Francis has peripheral IV for nutritional support. You discover that for the second time this shift, Francis has "removed" the IV. You would restrain Francis and restart a new IV as soon as possible.[a]	1	2	3	4	5	6
2. There is an order for blood cultures to be drawn if Francis's temperature goes above 104°F. You find that Francis's temperature is 103.9°F. Blood cultures should not be drawn.	1	2	3	4	5	6
3. You find that Francis's level of consciousness has decreased. You would initiate neuro checks every 2 hours.[a]	1	2	3	4	5	6
4. Francis has requested not to be weighed this morning. You would cancel this morning's weight.	1	2	3	4	5	6
5. Francis should be in an intensive care unit where close monitoring and one-to-one nursing care is available.[a]	1	2	3	4	5	6

6. Francis should not have aggressive care given.	1	2	3	4	5	6
7. Francis prefers the supine position only. You would turn this patient every 2 hours regardless.[a]	1	2	3	4	5	6
8. Vital signs should be taken at least every 2 hours.[a]	1	2	3	4	5	6
9. The need for comfort and rest is the primary concern.	1	2	3	4	5	6
10. A complete nursing assessment should be performed each shift.[a]	1	2	3	4	5	6
11. If Francis's respiratory status declines, chest physiotherapy and suctioning should be provided every 2 hours.[a]	1	2	3	4	5	6
12. Francis has continued to deteriorate and now needs supplemental nutritional support. The patient has needed the nasogastric tube replaced two times on your shift, and has just managed to pull out the third NG tube. You would leave the NG tube out.	1	2	3	4	5	6
13. Francis is not tolerating the tube feedings. The physician obtained a nutrition consultation and wants to begin TPN. TPN should not be started.	1	2	3	4	5	6

SOURCE: From "Aggressiveness of nursing care for older patients and those with do-not-resuscitate orders," by S. I. Shelley, R. M. Zahorchak, and C. D. S. Gambrill, 1987, Nursing Research, 36, pp. 157-162. Reprinted with permission.

[a] Item flipped for scoring.

Instrument 7.5b

Frank is a 32-year-old gay (homosexual) patient hospitalized with AIDS-related Pneumocystis carinii *pneumonia in your unit. After three weeks of aggressive antibiotic therapy, there has been no clinical improvement. Frank is lethargic, but easily aroused. Due to the poor prognosis of this case and at the request of the patient and family members, a Do-Not-Resuscitate order has been written.*

In questionnaires depicting the patient without a DNR order, the entire last sentence was replaced by the statement, "His prognosis is poor."

SOURCE: From "AIDS-related risk factors, medical diagnoses, do-not-resuscitate orders and aggressiveness of nursing care," by D. A. Forrester, 1990, *Nursing Research, 39,* pp. 350-354.

Instrument 7.5b

Francis is a 72-year-old patient with fulminating resistant-pseudomonas sepsis in your unit. After 3 weeks of aggressive antibiotic therapy, there has been no clinical improvement. Francis is lethargic but easily aroused. Because of the poor prognosis of this case and at the request of the patient and immediate family members, a Do-Not-Resuscitate order has been written.

The last sentence was eliminated in half the distributed questionnaires.

Appropriateness of Care Questionnaire

Item	Posited subscale
1. Francis has requested not to be weighed this morning. This morning's weight should be canceled.	Physical
2. Francis verbalizes the informed, rational desire to take his own life. He should not be prevented from doing so.	Psychosocial
3. Francis has continued to deteriorate and now needs supplemental nutritional support. The patient has needed the nasogastric tube replaced two times on your shift, and has just managed to pull out the third nasogastric tube. The nasogastric tube should be left out.	Physical
4. If Francis's respiratory status declines, chest physiotherapy and suctioning should not be provided every 2 hours.	Physical
5. Francis should be in an intensive care unit where close monitoring and one-to-one nursing care is available.	Physical
6. Francis has a peripheral IV for nutritional support. You discover that for the second time this shift, Francis has "removed" the IV. Francis should be restrained, and a new IV started as soon as possible.	Physical
7. You find that Francis's level of consciousness has decreased. Neuro checks should be initiated every 2 hours.	Physical

Item	Posited subscale
8. Francis is not tolerating the tube feedings. The physician obtained a nutrition consultation and wants to begin TPN. TPN should not be started.	Physical
9. There is an order for blood cultures to be drawn if Francis' temperature rises above 104°F. You find that Francis' temperature is 103.9°F. Blood cultures should not be drawn.	Physical
10. The issue of whether Francis would like to be discharged to a hospice or his home should be raised with him or his family.	Psychosocial
11. Vital signs should be taken at least every 2 hours.	Physical
12. Efforts should not be made to elicit Francis' feelings about his illness.	Psychosocial
13. Francis should not have aggressive care given.	Physical
14. Francis prefers the supine position only. He should be turned every 2 hours regardless.	Physical
15. Francis shows signs of anxiety. Anxiety-reducing medications and/or nonpharmacologic means (such as touch, presence) should be tried.	Psychosocial
16. Visits from immediate family and friends should be restricted.	Psychosocial
17. The need for comfort and rest is the primary concern.	Physical
18. A complete nursing assessment should be performed every shift.	Physical
19. Francis should be reoriented frequently to person, place, time, and sounds he hears.	Psychosocial
20. If you had another patient who was equally ill, your care of Francis would be affected.	

SOURCE: From "Critical care nurses' perceptions of appropriate care of the patient with orders not to resuscitate," by D. A. Sherman and K. Branum, 1995, *Heart and Lung, 24,* pp. 321-329. Reprinted with permission.

LEVEL OF MANAGEMENT IN NEONATAL CLINICAL SITUATIONS

Developed by Deborah A. Raines

INSTRUMENT DEVELOPMENT, ADMINISTRATION, AND SCORING

Neonatal nurses practice in an environment established on the expectation that high-technology neonatal intensive care units (NICUs) save and cure even the tiniest and sickest infants. Although NICUs have increased survival, questions have been raised about the usefulness and purpose of the interventions they offer (Raines, 1996).

The Level of Management in Neonatal Clinical Situations instrument consists of three clinical vignettes involving (a) a delivery room resuscitation of a very low birth weight infant, (b) management of an infant with a chromosomal anomaly, and (c) continuing care of a chronically ill infant. The two questions accompanying each vignette elicit the providers' degree of agreement or disagreement for three levels of management of the described infant—aggressive care, limited/conservative care, and comfort care—and the importance of items of information in influencing these choices (Raines, 1996).

PSYCHOMETRIC PROPERTIES

The vignettes used in this instrument are based on actual clinical situations reflecting the typology of infants previously reported in the literature. Judges certified in and expert in neonatal nursing and ethics supported content validity. Instrument testing was carried out with 356 neonatal nurses.

Internal consistency estimates of reliability for the scales ranged from .62 to .89. A principal components factor analysis of the information influences identified three subscales consistent with the conceptual model underlying the development of the instrument: (a) infant characteristics including birth weight, gestational age, and medical diagnosis, (b) family status (parents' marital and economic situation), and (c) unit/professional protocol, representing the external guidelines or rules that guide a nurse's practice behavior (Raines, 1996). This finding supports construct validity.

SUMMARY AND CRITIQUE

NICU nurses play a pivotal role in creating a forum in which consistent sensitive and knowledgeable decision making can occur as ethical questions emerge (Raines, 1994). Findings show that individual nurses have clearly defined preferences about treatment alternatives.

It should be noted that the instrument assumes that the parents' views are the same as those of the care providers and thus leaves unstudied those instances in which there are differences. Available data for this instrument show adequate initial psychometric characteristics, although improvement in reliability should be addressed, as should the testing of the sensitivity to intervention.

Most patient care is collaborative. Widely divergent and unacknowledged variation in practice choices can result in frustration and distress for individual practitioners and conflict between team members, which can ultimately have an adverse impact on the quality of patient care (Raines, 1996). This instrument should be helpful in exploring the extent of agreement with different degrees of management intensity and the factors influencing these choices.

REFERENCES

Raines, D. A. (1994). Values influencing neonatal nurses' perceptions and choices. *Western Journal of Nursing Research, 16*, 675-691.

Raines, D. A. (1996). Choices of neonatal nurses in ambiguous clinical situations. *Neonatal Network, 15*(1), 17-25.

Instrument 7.6

LEVEL OF MANAGEMENT IN
NEONATAL CLINICAL SITUATIONS

Directions: You will be presented with three situations representative of types of patients encountered in neonatal units. Please read each situation and answer the questions that follow. There are no right or wrong answers. The best answer is your own choice based on your nursing practice in the neonatal unit.

As you approach each situation, base your answers on the following assumptions:

1. The infant is a patient at the hospital where you work.
2. You are the infant's nurse.
3. The parent's views are the same as yours.

Situation 1

You are in the delivery room for the delivery of a 24-week gestation pregnancy. At birth, the infant is limp and has a heart rate of 110 bpm and a weak but spontaneous cry. You estimate that the infant weights between 450 and 500 gm. The eyes are fused, and the skin is thin and transparent.

Situation 2

An infant is brought to the nursery following a vaginal delivery at 35 weeks gestation. The infant exhibits characteristics of Trisomy-13, including rocker-bottom feet, low-set ears, cleft lip and palate, polydactyly, and clenched fists. The diagnosis of Trisomy-13 is confirmed by chromosomal analysis.

Situation 3

A 3 kg infant was born at 37.5 weeks gestation, secondary to placental abruptio. At birth, the infant was normal appearing, well nourished, limp without tone, and blue without spontaneous respirations. Resuscitation was initiated, and the infant was transferred to a medical center.

The infant is 45 days old. Pupils are fixed and dilated. The infant is spastic in all four extremities and requires continuous nasogastric feeding and cardiorespiratory support. The neurologist states that all movements are spinal in nature and there is little chance of long-term survival and no chance for functional development.

*Participants were asked to respond to the two
following questions for each of the above situations.*

1. The following are three levels of intervention available for the care and management of infants. Please **circle** the number that indicates your agreement with each alternative in the type of infant described in the above situation.

	Completely Disagree	Com-pletely Agree
Aggressive Care: Do everything possible to keep the infant alive. This may include but not be limited to initiation or continuation of mechanical ventilation, pharmacological support of vital functions, surgery, and other invasive interventions.	1 2 3 4 5 6 7	
Limited/Conservative Care: Care plan includes initiation and continuation of some treatments for the infant, which may include suctioning, noninvasive oxygen administration, and feedings, but does not include any invasive interventions such as intubation and mechanical ventilation or surgery.	1 2 3 4 5 6 7	
Comfort Care: Do not initiate or continue any treatments for the infant other than providing warmth and comfort.	1 2 3 4 5 6 7	

2. The following is a list of information that may influence your thinking about and your behavior in this type of situation. Please **circle** the number that indicates how important you feel each piece of information is to your behavior as a nurse in the care and management of the type of infant described in this situation.

	Least Important				Most Important		
Infant's gestational age	1	2	3	4	5	6	7
Opinion of consultants	1	2	3	4	5	6	7
Family's socioeconomic status	1	2	3	4	5	6	7
Current standards of care as defined by professional organizations	1	2	3	4	5	6	7
The Baby Doe regulations	1	2	3	4	5	6	7
Unit protocols	1	2	3	4	5	6	7
Expectations of physician	1	2	3	4	5	6	7
Infant's medical diagnosis	1	2	3	4	5	6	7
Results of diagnostic tests	1	2	3	4	5	6	7
Hospital philosophy or mission statement	1	2	3	4	5	6	7
Marital status of the parents	1	2	3	4	5	6	7
The ANA Code For Nurses	1	2	3	4	5	6	7
Infant's birth weight	1	2	3	4	5	6	7

Comments:

SOURCE: From "Choices of neonatal nurses in ambiguous clinical situations," by D. A. Raines, 1996, *Neonatal Network, 15*(1), pp. 17-25. Reprinted by permission of *Neonatal Network*.®

Moral Sensitivity

Moral sensitivity is the ability to identify an ethical problem and to understand the ethical consequences of the decisions made. More specifically, it involves building a trusting relationship with the patient and responding to his or her perceived needs, establishing moral meaning for decisions made, expressing a moral motivation to act in the best interest of the patient, and modifying the patient's autonomy when necessary. This construct emphasizes that moral decision making within a provider-patient relationship is not always deduced from rational thinking or the application of moral principles—it is also an emotive process, part of caring (Lutzen, Evertzon, & Nordin, 1997).

Moral sensitivity was derived from observation of practice and is believed to be important for an ethical practitioner, although the relationship between moral sensitivity and moral behavior (actions taken) has not yet been explicated. Moral sensitivity has been studied more often in nurses than in others because it is thought that these practitioners face the challenge of interpreting the moral demand as expressed by the patient and yet must act according to medical knowledge (Lutzen & Nordin, 1993).

REFERENCES

Lutzen, K., Evertzon, M., & Nordin, C. (1997). Moral sensitivity in psychiatric practice. *Nursing Ethics, 4*, 472-482.
Lutzen, K., & Nordin, C. (1993). Benevolence, a central moral concept derived from a grounded theory of nursing decision making in psychiatric settings. *Journal of Advanced Nursing, 18*, 1106-1111.

MORAL SENSITIVITY QUESTIONNAIRE (MSQ)

Developed by Kim Lutzen, Connie Nordin, and Gunilla Brolin

INSTRUMENT DEVELOPMENT, ADMINISTRATION, AND SCORING

Although other instruments have focused on cognitive aspects of moral decision making, the Moral Sensitivity Questionnaire (MSQ) is built on background studies of the experience of moral decision making in psychiatric nursing practice. In particular, it addresses the provider's manner of making sense of a perceived moral conflict and justifying "good" actions. Moral sensing is defined as a capacity for moral knowledge involving the integration of contextual knowledge, practical experience, intuition, and feeling a genuine motivation to do that which is for the patient's good. In the psychiatric nurses studied, a central dilemma was how to maintain a trusting relationship while following treatment principles with which the patient might not agree, therefore limiting the patient's self-choice (Lutzen & Nordin, 1993). Scores of individual items are summed.

PSYCHOMETRIC PROPERTIES

Because Lutzen, Nordin, and Brolin believe that hypothetical social dilemmas tend to separate moral problems from their contingencies, items were developed inductively from qualitative studies of actual practice. This should increase validity. Six experts reviewed the MSQ for content validity. Testing of the instrument with 79 psychiatric nurses provided a basis for scale revision that resulted in a Cronbach's alpha of .73 for the total scale. Administration to an additional population of 145 psychiatric nurses and 150 medical surgical nurses showed a Cronbach's alpha of .78 (Lutzen & Nordin, 1993).

Subsequent study with 754 psychiatrists showed a Cronbach's alpha of .64 (Lutzen & Schreiber, 1998).

Factor analysis confirmed six dimensions of moral sensitivity: interpersonal orientation, structural moral meaning, expressing benevolence, modifying autonomy, experiencing moral conflict, and trust in medical knowledge and principles of care (Lutzen, Nordstrom, & Evertzon, 1995).

SUMMARY AND CRITIQUE

The special moral responsibilities of psychiatric practice are central to the MSQ. Decisions about whether a patient has the cognitive and emotional capacity to be responsible for his or her own actions are primarily based on observations made within the practitioner-patient relationship. Consequent limitations on human freedom and dignity are perhaps particularly problematic in psychiatric practice. The moral domain in psychiatry is even more complex because of conflicting views about the etiology of mental illness, which is frequently not based on scientific facts but rather on different conceptions of normality (Lutzen & Nordin, 1993).

The MSQ has been used across disciplines to identify potential differences in the way in which ethical problems are viewed and may be used for this purpose within a practice team.

The finding of lower reliability of the scale with psychiatrists than with psychiatric nurses likely reflects that the instrument was developed using grounded theory observations of nursing practice. This discrepancy may indicate that nurses and physicians are sensitive to different types of problems encountered in daily practice (Lutzen, Evertzon, & Nordin, 1997).

The MSQ is one of the few instruments developed within a care ethic frame of reference. It views ethical conflicts as grounded in dynamic interpersonal interactions. Although there are few, if any, other instruments representing this perspective with which one could do validity studies, predictive validity could be tested, and sensitivity of the MSQ to interventions should be checked.

REFERENCES

Lutzen, K., Evertzon, M., & Nordin, C. (1997). Moral sensitivity in psychiatric practice. *Nursing Ethics, 4,* 472-482.

Lutzen, K., & Nordin, C. (1993). Structuring moral meaning in psychiatric nursing practice. *Scandinavian Journal of Caring Science, 7,* 175-180.

Lutzen, K., Nordstrom, G., & Evertzon, M. (1995). Moral sensitivity in nursing practice. *Scandinavian Journal of Caring Science, 9,* 131-138.

Lutzen, K., & Schreiber, R. (1998). Moral survival in a nontherapeutic environment. *Issues in Mental Health Nursing, 19,* 303-315.

Instrument 8.1

MORAL SENSITIVITY QUESTIONNAIRE
(TRANSLATION OF THE SWEDISH VERSION)*

1) It is my responsibility as a psychiatrist to have knowledge of the patient's total situation.

2) My work would feel meaningless if I never saw any improvement in my patients.

3) It is important that I should obtain a positive response from the patient in everything I do.

4) When I need to make a decision against the will of a patient, I do so according to my opinion about what is good care.

5) If I should lose the patient's trust I would feel that my work would lack meaning.

6) When I have to make difficult decisions for the patient, it is important always to be honest with him or her.

7) I believe that good psychiatric care includes respecting the patient's self-choice.

8) If a patient does not have insight into the illness, there is little I can do for him or her.

9) I am often confronted by situations in which I experience conflict in how to approach the patient.

10) I believe that it is important to have firm principles for the care of certain patients.

11) I often face situations in which it is difficult to know what action is ethically right for a particular patient.

12) If I am unacquainted with the case history of a patient, I follow the rules that are available.

13) What is most important in my psychiatric practice is my relationship with my patients.

14) I often face situations in which I have difficulty in allowing a patient to make his or her own decision.

15) I always base my actions on medical knowledge of what is the best treatment, even if the patient protests.

16) I think that good psychiatric care often includes making decisions *for* the patient.

17) I rely mostly on the nurses' knowledge about a patient when I am unsure.

18) Most of all, it is the reactions of patients that show me if I have made the right decision.

19) I often think about my own values and norms that may influence my actions.

20) My own experience is more useful than theory in situations in which it is difficult to know what is ethically right.

21) It is important that I should have rules to follow when a patient who is *not* being treated under the Mental Health Act refuses treatment.

22) I believe that good psychiatric care includes patient participation, even of those with serious mental disorders.

23) I am often caught in predicaments where I have to make decisions without the patient's participation.

24) If a patient is being treated under the Mental Health Act, I expect nursing staff to follow my orders even if the patient is noncompliant.

25) I find it difficult to give good psychiatric care against the will of the patient.

26) Sometimes there are good reasons to threaten a patient with an injection if an oral medication is refused.

27) In situations in which it is difficult to know what is right, I consult my colleagues about what should be done.

28) I rely mostly on my own feelings when I have to make a difficult decision for a patient.

29) As a psychiatrist, I must always know how individual patients on my ward should be respectfully approached.

30) I find meaning in my role even if I do not succeed in helping a patient to gain insight into his or her illness.

The anchors are:

1	2	3	4	5	6	7
completely agree					completely disagree	

SOURCE: From "Moral sensitivity in psychiatric practice," by K. Lutzen, M. Evertzon, and C. Nordin, 1997, *Nursing Ethics, 4,* pp. 472-482. © K. Lutzen 1995. Reprinted with kind permission of Arnold Publishers.

NOTE: *In other versions, "nurse" is used instead of "psychiatrist."

Ethical
Practice Environment

The ethical practice environment reflects the values operative in that milieu regarding such issues as the rights of patients and the moral agency of health care professionals. These values are reflected in the norms and expectations that are shared, to a greater or lesser extent, by employees, with a high degree of consensus reflecting a strong environment. The ethical environment is believed to affect the ability of providers to deliver care that meets ethical standards and to affect their satisfaction with their ability to live up to the expectations of their professional roles. The two instruments in this section were developed to describe how practitioners perceive their practice environments, and to evaluate efforts to improve the environment.

Challenges about ethics are inherent in and an expected part of professional practice. What registered nurses find problematic is health care practice that does not protect patients, that excludes nurses from participation in deliberations regarding their practice as it relates to ethics, and the absence of policies and administrators that support nurses' ability to practice ethically (McDaniel, 1998). Ethics work satisfaction is positively related to retention of workers and can be enhanced by administrators (McDaniel, 1995), something that is important in an age of significant and prolonged shortage of nurses.

REFERENCES

McDaniel, C. (1995). Organizational culture and ethics work satisfaction. *Journal of Nursing Administration, 25*(11), 15-21.

McDaniel, C. (1998). Ethical environment: Reports of practicing nurses. *Nursing Clinics of North America, 33*, 363-371.

ETHICS ENVIRONMENT QUESTIONNAIRE (EEQ)

Developed by Charlotte McDaniel

INSTRUMENT DEVELOPMENT, ADMINISTRATION, AND SCORING

Organizational culture is defined as the ways of thinking, behaving, and believing that members of a unit have in common, with a focus on behaviors reflected in norms and expectations shared by employees. Study has shown that in constructive cultures in which employees are encouraged to interact and approach tasks in positive ways, workers demonstrate higher job satisfaction, retention, and performance. The opposite is true in passive-defensive organizational culture situations. An important aspect of organizational culture for nurses is satisfaction with how the work environment supports positive management of their ethical concerns. Initial work by McDaniel (1995) showed a positive relationship between constructive culture and ethics work satisfaction.

The Ethics Environment Questionnaire (EEQ) is a 20-item self-administered questionnaire using a Likert-type 5-point format. Response choices are strongly agree (5), agree (4), undecided (3), disagree (2), and strongly disagree (1). Some items are worded negatively, thereby requiring scoring adjustment. McDaniel (1995) indicates that the EEQ can be used to measure the ethics environment across settings.

Reading level for the EEQ is ninth grade; mean administration time is 10 minutes. Item scores are summed and averaged to obtain an overall score, with scores of 3.5 (out of a possible 5) and above interpreted as a positive ethics environment. The scale has been tested with 450 volunteer RN respondents in acute care settings, showing a mean score of 3.1. Individual item scores may be found in McDaniel (1997).

PSYCHOMETRIC PROPERTIES

McDaniel indicates that items reflect a review of the literature and standards of organizations such as the Joint Commission for the Accreditation of Healthcare Organizations (JCAHO), and were tested and culled or retained. Content validity was judged acceptable by expert panels and by practitioners. Internal consistency (Cronbach's alpha) was .93 and test-retest reliability over a four-month period .88. Factor analysis showed the EEQ to be unidimensional (McDaniel, 1997).

In support of its validity, constructive organizational culture situations showed a significant positive relationship to the ethics subscale and passive-defensive cultures were negatively related to the ethics subscale. Scores on the EEQ and the Ability to Manage Disagreement Scale also showed the same correlation. In addition, respondents who reported strong retention in their work sites and were willing to recommend them had scores that strongly corresponded with positive scores for their ethics environment. A subscale of respondents who had little or no access to an institutional ethics committee had low scores (McDaniel, 1997). All of this evidence supports the instrument's validity.

Respondents who participated in an on-site ethics program showed significant changes in their EEQ scores that a control group did not show, lending support to the scale's sensitivity. Respondents with self-reported ethical dilemmas or difficulties showed low EEQ scores (McDaniel, 1997). All of these relationships are in the expected direction.

SUMMARY AND CRITIQUE

The EEQ is used to measure the opinions of health care providers about ethics in their clinical practice organizations. Practice settings in which professional nurses could approach other employees and tasks in ways to enhance their own satisfaction needs and to resolve problems were associated with inclusion in ethics decisions, fewer reported "problems" from ethics issues, and ability to resolve disagreements between professional groups (McDaniel, 1997).

Associations accrediting health care organizations now include standards related to ethics. The EEQ could help document staff perceptions of organizational support for conducting ethical aspects of professional practice and for identifying units for which additional support for staff is necessary. When new strategies, structures, or processes regarding ethics are introduced, it is important to evaluate their effect on the ethics environment as perceived by practitioners. With additional experience with the EEQ, score interpretation will be enhanced. Although the instrument is intended for use with various health professionals and sites, to date it has predominantly been used with registered nurses in acute care hospitals (McDaniel, 1997).

REFERENCES

McDaniel, C. (1995). Organizational culture and ethics work satisfaction. *Journal of Nursing Administration, 25*(11), 15-21.

McDaniel, C. (1997). Development and psychometric properties of the Ethics Environment Questionnaire. *Medical Care, 9,* 901-914.

HOSPITAL ETHICAL CLIMATE SURVEY (HECS)

Developed by Linda L. Olson

INSTRUMENT DEVELOPMENT, ADMINISTRATION, AND SCORING

The ethical climate of an organization, as perceived by a group of its workers, is believed to affect ethical practice, job satisfaction, and quality of care. It can be viewed as a set of institutional practices and assessed by measuring how decisions having ethical content are solved, the presence of organizational conditions that allows employees to engage in ethical reflection, or both. These include the option to disagree with one another, inclusion of those with a stake in the decision, access to information to make informed decisions, and encouragement of questioning and debate (Olson, 1998).

Items are organized according to the relationships of peers, patients, managers, the hospital, and physicians and are rated on a 5-point scale from 1 (almost never true) to 5 (almost always true). A mean score is obtained for the instrument as a whole as well as for individual factors (Olson, 1998).

PSYCHOMETRIC PROPERTIES

Conditions for ethical reflection and findings from business and nursing ethics studies were sources of items. Content validity was supported by a concept analysis of ethical climate and judgment of seven nurses expert in ethics, organizational climate, and nursing administration. The HECS was pretested for clarity. It was then administered to 360 RNs in clinical practice at two acute care hospitals in one midwestern city (Olson, 1998).

Construct validity was supported by findings of the relationship of the HECS with another instrument, the Integrity Audit. The two hospitals in which the nurses were employed had different organizational characteristics (religious affiliation and for-profit ownership) and showed differences that might be expected (known groups technique). Five factors were found with Cronbach's alphas as follows: relationship of nurses with peers (.73), patients (.68), managers (.92), hospital (.77), and physicians (.81), with .91 representing the total instrument. Analysis shows that the subscales cannot be considered to be independent and so must be perceived only as a method to organize the items comprising the measure of ethical climate (Olson, 1998).

SUMMARY AND CRITIQUE

The HECS has acceptable initial reliability and validity. Future work is needed to test the instrument in various health care organizations and to determine whether it is useful for diagnostic and evaluative purposes (Olson, 1998) and sensitive to intervention. Its potential usefulness is in assessing the ethical environment for nursing practice and the impact of mechanisms and programs to support that environment (Olson, 1998).

REFERENCE

Olson, L. L. (1998). Hospital nurses' perceptions of the ethical climate of their work setting. *Image, 30,* 345-349.

Instrument 9.2

HOSPITAL ETHICAL
CLIMATE SURVEY

Directions: Here is a series of statements relating to various practices within your work setting. Please respond in terms of how it is in your current job on your current unit. As you read and respond to each statement, think of some difficult patient care issues you have faced. For those items that refer to your manager, think of your immediate manager (nurse manager, assistant nurse manager, shift supervisor). It is important that you respond in terms of how it really is on your unit, not how you would prefer it to be. It is essential to answer every item. There are no right or wrong answers, so please respond honestly. Remember, all your responses will remain anonymous.

Please read each of the following statements. Then, circle one of the numbers on each line to indicate your response.

	Almost Never True	Seldom True	Sometimes True	Often True	Almost Always True
1. My peers listen to my concerns about patient care	1	2	3	4	5
2. Patients know what to expect from their care	1	2	3	4	5
3. When I'm unable to decide what's right or wrong in a patient care situation, my manager helps me	1	2	3	4	5
4. Hospital policies help me with difficult patient care issues/problems	1	2	3	4	5
5. Nurses and physicians trust one another	1	2	3	4	5
6. Nurses have access to the information necessary to solve a patient care issue/problem	1	2	3	4	5

	Almost Never True	Seldom True	Sometimes True	Often True	Almost Always True
7. My manager supports me in my decisions about patient care	1	2	3	4	5
8. A clear sense of the hospital's mission is shared with nurses	1	2	3	4	5
9. Physicians ask nurses for their opinions about treatment decisions	1	2	3	4	5
10. My peers help me with difficult patient care issues/problems	1	2	3	4	5
11. Nurses use the information necessary to solve a patient care issue/problem	1	2	3	4	5
12. My manager listens to me talk about patient care issues/ problems	1	2	3	4	5
13. The feelings and values of all parties involved in a patient care issue/problem are taken into account when choosing a course of action	1	2	3	4	5
14. I participate in treatment decisions for my patients	1	2	3	4	5
15. My manager is someone I can trust	1	2	3	4	5
16. Conflict is openly dealt with, not avoided	1	2	3	4	5
17. Nurses and physicians here respect each others' opinions, even when they disagree about what is best for patients	1	2	3	4	5

	Almost Never True	Seldom True	Sometimes True	Often True	Almost Always True
18. I work with competent colleagues	1	2	3	4	5
19. The patient's wishes are respected	1	2	3	4	5
20. When my peers are unable to decide what's right or wrong in a particular patient care situation, I have observed that my manager helps them	1	2	3	4	5
21. There is a sense of questioning, learning, and seeking creative responses to patient care problems	1	2	3	4	5
22. Nurses and physicians respect one another	1	2	3	4	5
23. Safe patient care is given on my unit	1	2	3	4	5
24. My manager is someone I respect	1	2	3	4	5
25. I am able to practice nursing on my unit as I believe it should be practiced	1	2	3	4	5
26. Nurses are supported and respected in this hospital	1	2	3	4	5

Factor 1 (Peers): Items 1, 10, 18, 23

Factor 2 (Patients): Items 2, 6, 11, 19

Factor 3 (Managers): Items 3, 7, 12, 15, 20, 24

Factor 4 (Hospital): Items 4, 8, 13, 25

Factor 5 (Physicians): Items 5, 9, 14, 17, 22, 26

BACKGROUND DATA

Directions: These questions concern the backgrounds of those who respond to this survey. As with all answers to this survey, your responses will be kept confidential. Please circle the appropriate number or fill in the blank.

1. Are you?
   Female   1
   Male   2
2. In what year were you born? 19_____
3. What is your basic nursing education?
   Associate degree   1
   Diploma   2
   Baccalaureate (Nursing)   3
   Baccalaureate (Other field)   4
   Year completed 19_____
4. What is your highest degree earned?
   Associate degree   1
   Diploma   2
   Baccalaureate (Nursing)   3
   Baccalaureate (Other field)   4
   Master's (Nursing)   5
   Master's (Other field)   6
   Doctoral Degree (Nursing)   7
   Doctoral Degree   8
5. How long have you worked as a Registered Nurse?
   _____ Years   _____ Months
6. How long have you been employed at your present hospital?
   _____ Years   _____ Months
7. What is your present nursing position?
   Staff nurse   1
   Assistant head nurse   2
   Clinical specialist   3
   Other (please specify)   4
   _____
8. What is your race?
   African-American   1
   Caucasian   2
   Hispanic or Latino   3
   Asian or Pacific Islander   4
   American Indian   5
   Other (please specify)   6
   _____

SOURCE: From "Hospital nurses' perceptions of the ethical climate of their work setting," by L. L. Olson, 1998, *Image, 30,* 345-349. Reprinted with permission.

10 Recipient Selection

How to best allocate finite health care resources has become a major focus of health policy. A shortage of organs and tissues for transplantation has been present throughout most of the history of transplantation and is expected to worsen as transplantation becomes more successful and is offered to sicker and older patients. Fair distribution of health resources is essential to an ethical health care system. Currently, organ transplantation is the most extensive program requiring allocation of scarce resources.

No universal criteria have been established to allocate human organs for transplant, and various outcomes from transplant are valued differently—survival, quality of life, symptom frequency and distress, number of rejection episodes (Corley, Huff, Sayles, & Short, 1995). Although there seems to be some consensus on the unacceptability of social worth as a criterion for fair distribution, less consensus exists on the use of physical standards such as the presence of various disease states and psychosocial criteria such as health behavior and lifestyle issues.

The instrument in this section should help to describe differences in perspective. Yet to be developed are studies establishing the reliability with which criteria are applied to patients, and the relationship of selection criteria to medical and functional outcomes.

REFERENCE

Corley, M. C., Huff, S., Sayles, L., & Short, L. (1995). Patient and nurse criteria for heart transplant candidacy. *Medsurg Nursing, 4,* 211-215.

CRITERIA FOR SELECTION OF TRANSPLANT RECIPIENT SCALE (CSTR)

Developed by Mary C. Corley, Norman Westerberg,
R. K. Elswick, Jr., Dennis Connell, Janice Neil,
Gilda Sneed, and Vianna Witcher

INSTRUMENT DEVELOPMENT, ADMINISTRATION, AND SCORING

Criteria for decisions made for allocating scarce health care resources have obvious implications for issues of justice. In addition to the United Network for Organ Sharing (UNOS), criteria related to medical need, geographical distance from transplant center, waiting time, and other issues affect allocation decisions. Many transplant programs are confronted by other ethical concerns related to allocation. These include providing organs to patients who have high social profiles but do not meet UNOS criteria, patients who are hospitalized to keep them high on the UNOS waiting list or to control alcohol intake prior to transplant, or those who cannot pay for the transplant procedure. Furthermore, there is lack of agreement on whether addictive behaviors are of the candidate's making and therefore should affect selection for transplant, on how benefit is defined both for the candidate and for society, and on whether age and social network affect survival or are unfair selection criteria (Corley et al., 1998).

The major ethical argument for employing psychosocial criteria in the selection of those to receive transplants is the same as for medical criteria—to allocate scarce organs and expensive care and technology to those patients likely to derive maximum benefit and longevity. The problem with using such criteria is that they may be confused with judgments of an individual's social worth, which are not regarded by most as acceptable grounds for choosing candidates (Olbrisch &

Levenson, 1995). If they are to be used, they must be applied with high validity and consistency (reliability).

The Criteria for Selection of Transplant Recipients Scale (CSTR) was adapted from the index developed by Olbrisch & Levenson (1991), which was in turn developed from criteria published by several transplant centers. This modified instrument lists lifestyle and psychosocial criteria that might be used for organ recipient selection. Responses are exclude (1), probably exclude (2), probably include (3), and include (4).

PSYCHOMETRIC PROPERTIES

The CSTR index was reviewed for content validity by 18 members of the North American Transplant Coordinators research committee and by three nurse experts in organ transplantation. After revisions, items receiving more than 90% agreement on the content validity index were included. The test-retest reliability of a nurse sample during a 3-week interval was .85. Through factor analysis, six factors were identified: current lifestyle/psychiatric problems, family/socioeconomic issues, habits, controlled lifestyle/psychiatric issues, cost, and stigmatized conditions. Details of the factor analysis may be found in Corley et al. (1998).

Use of the CSTR with patients and nurses found significantly different opinions for 71% of the criteria, with nurses more likely to identify reasons for exclusion (Corley, Huff, Sayles, & Short, 1995).

SUMMARY AND CRITIQUE

Basic philosophical and empirical questions about the criteria remain. Are they weighted equally or are some more important than others? Are criteria considered absolute or additive (candidate turned down for an accumulation of problems)? Perhaps of greatest concern is that actual data regarding the validity of psychosocial criteria used to predict transplant outcomes are very limited (Olbrisch & Levenson, 1995).

Patients who were in prison for a serious crime, used cocaine, had AIDS, or were HIV positive (criteria making up the stigma factor) were more likely to be labeled for exclusion from transplant than were those with other psychosocial/lifestyle characteristics. When transplant coordinators perceived that patients' psychosocial and lifestyle problems were under control or corrected, they were more likely to consider them for a transplant. For all but the cost factor, criteria were most stringent for heart transplants (Corley et al., 1998).

The CSTR Scale is useful for studying degree of consensus among transplant programs, based on the criteria that might be used to allocate organs. In their international study of transplant programs, Olbrisch and Levenson (1991) and Levenson and Olbrisch (1993) found that more than 70% of the programs would exclude patients for heart transplant on the basis of active schizophrenia, current suicidal state, history of multiple suicide attempts, dementia, severe mental retardation, or current substance abuse. There was less agreement on whether cigarette smoking, obesity, recent drug/alcohol abuse, criminality, personality disorder, mild mental retardation, controlled schizophrenia, and affective disorders would influence patient selection. Although a number of researchers have studied the effects of lifestyle and psychosocial characteristics on transplant patient outcomes, the findings are not conclusive (Corley & Sneed, 1994). The concern is that psychosocial factors predictive of survival may be confused with judgments of an individual's social worth and may be applied inconsistently (Olbrisch & Levenson, 1991).

The current version of the CSTR Scale has apparently not been used with transplant surgeons. In addition, issues of weight to be attached to criteria are not addressed. Studies that demonstrate the relationship of selection criteria to medical and functional outcomes are also needed, and the current instrument also does not address how psychosocial factors can be evaluated in a reproducible and consistent manner (Levenson & Olbrisch, 1993).

REFERENCES

Corley, M. C., Huff, S., Sayles, L., & Short, L. (1995). Patient and nurse criteria for heart transplant candidacy. *Medsurg Nursing, 4,* 211-215.

Corley, M. C., & Sneed, G. (1994). Criteria in the selection of organ transplant recipients. *Heart and Lung, 23,* 446-457.

Corley, M. C., Westerberg, N., Elswick, R. K., Jr., Connell, D., Neil, J., Sneed, G., & Witcher, V. (1998). Rationing organs using psychosocial and lifestyle criteria. *Research in Nursing and Health, 21,* 327-337.

Levenson, J. L., & Olbrisch, M. E. (1993). Psychosocial evaluation of organ transplant candidates. *Psychosomatics, 34,* 314-323.

Olbrisch, M. E., & Levenson, J. L. (1991). Psychosocial evaluation of heart transplant candidates: An international survey of process, criteria and outcomes. *Journal of Heart and Lung Transplantation, 10,* 948-955.

Olbrisch, M. E., & Levenson, J. L. (1995). Psychosocial assessment of organ transplant candidates. *Psychosomatics, 36,* 236-243.

Instrument 10.1

TRANSPLANT CRITERIA

Examine the characteristics on the left, and indicate whether that patient should be excluded or allowed to receive a transplant in the United States. (Circle appropriate number from 1 to 4)

> 1 = **EXCLUDE** from getting transplant (E)
> 2 = **PROBABLY EXCLUDE** (PE)
> 3 = **PROBABLY ALLOW** to get transplant (PA)
> 4 = **ALLOW** to get transplant (A)

		E	PE	PA	A
1.	Citizen of another country.	1	2	3	4
2.	Resident of a state other than where transplant is to be done.	1	2	3	4
3.	Patient has no family/friend for assistance after hospital discharge.	1	2	3	4
4.	Patient has experienced recent death or loss of a loved one.	1	2	3	4
5.	Patient is in prison for a serious crime.	1	2	3	4
6.	Patient has psychiatric problems and refuses to get treatment.	1	2	3	4
7.	Patient has had psychiatric problems, but was treated, and is now stable.	1	2	3	4
8.	Patient is quite depressed.	1	2	3	4
9.	Patient has been treated for depression in the past, but is not depressed at the present.	1	2	3	4
10.	Patient recently attempted suicide.	1	2	3	4
11.	Patient tried to commit suicide 10 years ago.	1	2	3	4
12.	Patient has tried to commit suicide several times, the most recent 6 months ago.	1	2	3	4
13.	Patient has tried to commit suicide while in the hospital awaiting transplant.	1	2	3	4
14.	Patient is not in touch with reality (confused).	1	2	3	4
15.	Patient is a pathological liar.	1	2	3	4
16.	Patient is mentally retarded with a 3rd grade level of thinking.	1	2	3	4

	E	PE	PA	A
17. Patient is mentally retarded and cannot take care of daily needs (feeding, toilet) without assistance.	1	2	3	4
18. Patient smokes.	1	2	3	4
19. Patient smoked, but quit when hospitalized.	1	2	3	4
20. Patient smokes a pipe, cigars or chews tobacco.	1	2	3	4
21. Patient is an alcoholic and gets drunk nearly every day.	1	2	3	4
22. Patient is a recovering alcoholic, and has not had a drink in 6 months.	1	2	3	4
23. Patient uses cocaine or heroin.	1	2	3	4
24. Patient uses marijuana.	1	2	3	4
25. Patient used, but not longer uses, cocaine or heroin.	1	2	3	4
26. Patient no longer uses marijuana.	1	2	3	4
27. Although patient has quit smoking, drinking or using drugs, organ failure was directly linked to use of alcohol, smoking or drug use.	1	2	3	4
28. Patient is more than 40% above ideal weight.	1	2	3	4
29. Patient is overweight by 15 pounds.	1	2	3	4
30. Patient states he/she has tried a prescribed diet, but cannot follow one.	1	2	3	4
31. Patient has a history of not taking prescription medications correctly.	1	2	3	4
32. Patient comes from a troubled family.	1	2	3	4
33. Patient has AIDS.	1	2	3	4
34. Patient is HIV positive.	1	2	3	4
35. Patient does not understand what the transplant procedure involves.	1	2	3	4
36. Patient probably won't follow the doctor's orders after transplant (did not follow doctor's prescribed treatment as illness progressed).	1	2	3	4
37. Patient lives alone.	1	2	3	4
38. Patient was not employed prior to becoming ill.	1	2	3	4
39. Patient does not plan to return to work after transplant, even if transplant is successful.	1	2	3	4

		E	PE	PA	A
40.	Patient has no insurance that would cover the cost of the transplant procedure.	1	2	3	4
41.	Patient cannot pay for the transplant procedure.	1	2	3	4
42.	Patient's health care is covered by Medicaid.	1	2	3	4
43.	Enough donations have been collected to pay for the transplant, but the patient cannot afford the expensive medication necessary for the rest of his/her life.	1	2	3	4
44.	Patient's chance of living through surgery is less than 10%, but transplant is the only hope. This transplant deprives another good (well-matched) patient from receiving the organ.	1	2	3	4
45.	Patient cannot pay for immunosuppressive medication after transplant.	1	2	3	4
46.	Patient is actively involved in substance abuse program.	1	2	3	4
47.	Patient is openly hostile to staff.	1	2	3	4

48. Do you believe that there should be an age limit to receive an organ transplant? Yes_____ No_____

49. If yes, what should be the upper age limit? _____
    If yes, what upper age limit? _____

SOURCE: From "Rationing organs using psychosocial and lifestyle criteria," by M. C. Corley, N. Westerberg, R. K. Elswick, Jr., D. Connell, J. Neil, G. Sneed, and V. Witcher, 1998, *Research in Nursing and Health, 21,* pp. 327-337. Copyright ©1998 by John Wiley & Sons, Inc. Reprinted by permission of John Wiley & Sons, Inc.

Instrument 10.2

Table 2. Factor Loadings for Indicators of Psychosocial and Lifestyle Criteria for Selecting Transplant Recipients (*N* = 559)

Variable	Factor					
	1	2	3	4	5	6
Current						
Does not understand transplant procedures.	.66	−.01	.11	−.01	.13	−.09
Probably won't follow physician's orders after transplant.	.63	.12	.22	.03	.09	.05
History of not taking prescription medications correctly.	.61	.20	.16	.09	.07	−.08
Psychiatric problems and refuses treatment.	.61	.11	.14	.00	.09	.21
Recently attempted suicide.	.61	.07	−.08	.30	.05	.22
Tried to commit suicide while in hospital awaiting transplant.	.58	.07	−.06	.01	−.08	.22
Pathological liar.	.54	.16	.23	.08	.07	.14
Quite depressed.	.53	.22	−.19	.28	−.07	.09
Tried to commit suicide several times, as recently as 6 months ago	.51	.11	.07	.20	.00	.32
Not in touch with reality (confused).	.50	−.19	.03	.31	.11	.02
Open hostility to staff.	.47	.18	.18	.17	.19	.06
Weight is more than 40% above ideal weight.	.42	.16	.21	.26	.23	−.20
Tried but cannot follow prescribed diet.	.33	.32	.32	.22	.11	−.17
Family/Socioeconomic						
Lives alone.	.04	.71	.19	.03	.02	.09
Not employed prior to becoming ill.	.01	.70	.20	.09	.13	−.06
Does not plan to return to work after transplant, even if transplant is successful.	.06	.65	.17	.08	.11	−.09
Comes from a troubled family.	.21	.60	.11	.08	.10	.08
No family/friend for assistance after discharge.	.19	.57	.17	−.12	.12	.20
Experienced death or loss of loved one.	.18	.39	−.17	.18	.04	.05
Mentally retarded with a third-grade level of thinking.	.21	.38	.29	.18	.07	.20
Health care is covered by Medicaid.	−.03	.38	.12	.12	.23	−.03
Overweight by 15 pounds.	.15	.38	.12	.28	.00	−.19
Mentally retarded and can't take care of daily needs (feeding, toilet) without assistance.	.25	.33	.33	.06	.08	.21
Habits						
Smoker.	.15	.17	.83	.21	−.07	.07
Smokes a pipe, cigars, or chews tobacco.	.14	.16	.81	.22	−.07	.06
Smoker, but quit when hospitalized.	.10	.18	.73	.27	−.05	.03

Variable	Factor					
	1	2	3	4	5	6
Marijuana user.	.16	.24	<u>.56</u>	.09	−.03	.12
Alcoholic and drinks nearly every day.	.38	.05	<u>.39</u>	−.06	.03	.32
Recover						
Recovering alcoholic and has not had a drink in 6 months.	.09	.08	.18	<u>.63</u>	.08	.08
No longer uses cocaine or heroin.	.12	.24	.30	<u>.60</u>	−.05	.22
Tried to commit suicide 10 years ago.	.20	.35	.03	<u>.58</u>	−.01	.10
Treated for depression in the past, not depressed at present.	.14	.47	−.13	<u>.55</u>	−.09	.19
Quit smoking, drinking, or using drugs; organ failure was directly linked to use of alcohol, smoking, or drugs.	.14	.03	.20	<u>.56</u>	.09	−.11
No longer uses marijuana.	−.07	.32	.39	<u>.51</u>	.03	.04
Actively involved in substance abuse program.	.16	−.13	.12	<u>.51</u>	.15	.09
Had psychiatric problems, was treated, and is now stable.	.09	.43	.02	<u>.49</u>	−.07	.22
Cost						
No insurance that would cover the cost of the transplant procedure.	.02	.14	−.03	−.03	<u>.85</u>	.15
Cannot pay for the transplant procedure.	.03	.13	−.04	−.05	<u>.85</u>	.16
Donations have been collected to pay for the transplant, but expensive medication necessary for the rest of his/her life is unaffordable.	.20	.13	.06	.19	<u>.78</u>	−.03
Cannot pay for immunosuppressive medication after the transplant.	.25	.10	−.03	.10	<u>.76</u>	−.02
Stigma						
Has AIDS.	.07	.01	.05	.07	.05	<u>.69</u>
HIV positive.	.08	.02	.02	.14	.08	<u>.61</u>
In prison for serious crime.	.27	.19	.16	.11	.08	<u>.48</u>
Cocaine or heroin user.	.37	−.04	.28	−.02	.00	<u>.45</u>
Eigenvalue	9.79	3.19	2.76	1.99	1.78	1.63
Variability[a]	22.2	7.3	6.3	4.5	4.1	3.7
M	1.90	3.34	2.51	2.60	3.09	1.29
SD	0.42	0.36	0.70	0.76	0.41	0.35
Cronbach's alpha	0.68	0.68	0.71	0.77	0.69	0.72

SOURCE: From "Rationing organs using psychosocial and lifestyle criteria," by M. C. Corley, N. Westerberg, R. K. Elswick, Jr., D. Connell, J. Neil, G. Sneed, and V. Witcher, 1998, *Research in Nursing and Health, 21*, pp. 327-337. Copyright ©1998 by John Wiley & Sons, Inc. Reprinted by permission of John Wiley & Sons, Inc.

[a]48% variability explained.

11

General Issues
for Health Professionals

This section presents two instruments that address macro-processes relevant to clinical ethics. One is used to study the consistency of recommendations of ethics in health care settings and the degree to which they conform to consensus statements and guidelines. Of course, variability in ethics advice is open to a number of meanings.

Instrument 11.2 addresses beliefs about the ethical issues involved in macro-allocation decisions that undergird health policy. This instrument, which is the only one on this topic that could be located, has been used to study the conflict in values between particular forms of rationing and the basic moral tenets of health professions. Because public policy sets the context in which health professionals practice, these kinds of conflicts frequently support ethical issues in clinical settings. Policies increasingly limit the amount of discretion clinicians have to exercise their moral judgment.

ETHICS CONSULTANTS' RECOMMENDATIONS (ECR)

Developed by Ellen Fox and Carol Stocking

INSTRUMENT DEVELOPMENT, ADMINISTRATION, AND SCORING

This instrument was developed to study the consistency of various ethics consultants' recommendations when they were presented with identical clinical information, and the conformity of these recommendations to well-known consensus statements and guidelines. The ability to obtain such a measurement is viewed as important to developing standards for evaluation of ethics consultation.

The Ethics Consultants' Recommendations (ECR) focuses on life-prolonging treatment, more specifically for patients in persistent vegetative state (PVS). The first part presents a hypothetical case with eight variations according to whether patients' prior wishes were known, whether family or friends were available, and the content of the AD and family wishes. Five responses are provided (Fox & Stocking, 1993).

Fox and Stocking note that life-prolonging treatment decisions were chosen because these are the most commonly raised issues for ethics consultants and guidelines for dealing with the issues have been endorsed. PVS was chosen because many of the subjective determinations that typically complicate ethics consultation are absent from PVS cases—decision-making capacity is not at issue, prognosis is known with considerable certainty, the condition is relatively well defined and consistent from case to case, the patient's situation is generally static, and quality of life assessments become irrelevant. Several sets of ethical guidelines are devoted exclusively to the condition (Fox & Stocking, 1993).

The ECR can be completed in 15 minutes. An intensity of life-prolonging treatment score is calculated by assigning scores of 1 to 4 for the ordered responses A to D and then summing responses across the seven vignettes. Higher scores represent more intensive treatment. Scores and discussion of their implications may be found in Fox and Stocking (1993).

PSYCHOMETRIC PROPERTIES

The ECR was administered to 154 attendees at an annual bioethics meeting. No evidence for judging the face or content validity or reliability of rater responses across time could be located for the ECR. Validity in the use of vignettes is best addressed through literature review, submission to experts including community members, and pretesting (Flaskerud, 1979). None of these activities could be located. Presumably such activities would strengthen but not overcome the inherent problem of using a static case with limited context as a proxy for live clinical situations.

SUMMARY AND CRITIQUE

Developers of the ECR found considerable variability in ethics consultants' recommendations for most of the hypothetical patients with PVS. There was general agreement between respondents for only one of the seven vignettes—the case of a person whose AD and family agreed that life-prolonging therapy be stopped. Although patient wishes were an important factor influencing recommendations, none of the respondents adhered invariably to the patients' AD. Analysis of existing guidelines showed lack of clear standards for any but the simplest of the hypotheticals and so were too equivocal to be useful for evaluating ethics consultants' recommendations. In addition, an "appropriate" level of agreement among ethics consultants has not been established, with some authors suggesting that a demonstration of a range of ethically acceptable alternatives should be the goal (Fox & Stocking, 1993).

Fox and Stocking raise very important issues about consistency in ethics consultants' recommendations. It will be important to formally establish content validity, to study relationships between responses on the ECR and real cases, and intrarater reliability across time. It will also be important to understand in detail the reasons underlying the inconsistent responses and to test the hypothesis of consistency in the numerous other content areas in which ethics consultants provide recommendations. This is perhaps particularly important in a content area in which the guidelines are more explicit, providing a standard against which to understand variation in consultants' recommendations.

REFERENCES

Flaskerud, J. H. (1979). Use of vignettes to elicit responses toward broad concepts. *Nursing Research, 28,* 210-212.

Fox, E., & Stocking, C. (1993). Ethics consultants' recommendations for life-prolonging treatment of patients in a persistent vegetative state. *Journal of the American Medical Association, 270,* 2578-2582.

Instrument 11.1

This questionnaire consists of eight variations on a clinical case. For each variation, please circle the letter corresponding to the single option which best describes what you would recommend if you were the ethics consultant on the case.

THE CLINICAL CASE:

You are consulted about limiting treatment for an unconscious patient who, in the opinion of the attending physician, a neurologist, and multiple other consultants, has virtually no chance of ever regaining consciousness and no known awareness of the outside world. Currently the only treatments the patient is receiving are fluid and nutrition through artificial means and routine nursing care; the patient does not require any other life-prolonging treatments (e.g., mechanical ventilation, antibiotics, etc.).

Variation #1: The patient described above left an advance directive which clearly and convincingly states that, in the event of a permanently unconscious and unaware state, the patient *did not want to be kept alive*. All family members *agree* with the patient's previously stated wishes and ask that all life-prolonging treatments, including artificial fluid and nutrition, be stopped. You recommend:

A   Continue routine nursing care but stop all treatments necessary for prolonging life, including artificial fluid and nutrition.

B   Continue fluid and nutrition through artificial means as well as routine nursing care, but do not add any additional procedures or treatments.

C   Continue fluid and nutrition through artificial means as well as routine nursing care, and in addition add the following procedures or treatments if they become necessary for prolonging life (circle as many numbers as apply):

> antibiotics . . . 1
> simple diagnostic tests . . . 2
> invasive diagnostic tests . . . 3
> blood or blood product transfusions . . . 4
> transfer to intensive care unit . . . 5
> dialysis . . . 6
> chemotherapy for cancer . . . 7
> minor surgery . . . 8
> major surgery . . . 9
> mechanical ventilation . . . 10
> cardiopulmonary resuscitation . . . 11
> organ transplantation . . . 12

D   Do everything possible to prolong life, including but not limited to the procedures and treatments listed in C.

E   Other (specify) _____

Please explain or qualify your recommendation:

_____

_____

_____

_____

If all legal and bureaucratic constraints were removed, would your recommendation change?

        YES . . . 1   NO . . . 2

If yes, in what way?

_____

_____

_____

_____

Variation #2: The patient described above left an advance directive which clearly and convincingly states that, in the event of a permanently unconscious and unaware state, the patient *did not want to be kept alive*. All family members *disagree* with the patient's previously stated wishes and ask that "everything possible" be done to prolong life. You recommend:

A   Continue routine nursing care but stop all treatments necessary for prolonging life, including artificial fluid and nutrition.

B   Continue fluid and nutrition through artificial means as well as routine nursing care, but do not add any additional procedures or treatments.

C   Continue fluid and nutrition through artificial means as well as routine nursing care, and in addition add the following procedures or treatments if they become necessary for prolonging life (circle as many numbers as apply):

        antibiotics . . . 1
        simple diagnostic tests . . . 2
        invasive diagnostic tests . . . 3
        blood or blood product transfusions . . . 4
        transfer to intensive care unit . . . 5
        dialysis . . . 6
        chemotherapy for cancer . . . 7
        minor surgery . . . 8
        major surgery . . . 9
        mechanical ventilation . . . 10
        cardiopulmonary resuscitation . . . 11
        organ transplantation . . . 12

D   Do everything possible to prolong life, including but not limited to the procedures and treatments listed in C.

E   Other (specify) _____

Please explain or qualify your recommendation:

_____
_____
_____
_____

If all legal and bureaucratic constraints were removed, would your recommendation change?

          YES . . . 1   NO . . . 2

If yes, in what way?

_____
_____
_____
_____

Variation #3: The patient described above left an advance directive which clearly and convincingly states that, in the event of a permanently unconscious and unaware state, the patient *wanted to be kept alive* as long as possible. All family members *agree* with the patient's previously stated wishes and ask that "everything possible" be done to prolong life. You recommend:

A   Continue routine nursing care but stop all treatments necessary for prolonging life, including artificial fluid and nutrition.

B   Continue fluid and nutrition through artificial means as well as routine nursing care, but do not add any additional procedures or treatments.

C   Continue fluid and nutrition through artificial means as well as routine nursing care, and in addition add the following procedures or treatments if they become necessary for prolonging life (circle as many numbers as apply):

          antibiotics . . . 1
          simple diagnostic tests . . . 2
          invasive diagnostic tests . . . 3
          blood or blood product transfusions . . . 4
          transfer to intensive care unit . . . 5
          dialysis . . . 6
          chemotherapy for cancer . . . 7
          minor surgery . . . 8
          major surgery . . . 9
          mechanical ventilation . . . 10
          cardiopulmonary resuscitation . . . 11
          organ transplantation . . . 12

D   Do everything possible to prolong life, including but not limited to the procedures and treatments listed in C.

E   Other (specify) _____

Please explain or qualify your recommendation:

_____
_____
_____
_____

If all legal and bureaucratic constraints were removed, would your recommendation change?

          YES . . . 1   NO . . . 2

If yes, in what way?

_____
_____
_____
_____

Variation #4: The patient described above left an advance directive which clearly and convincingly states that, in the event of a permanently unconscious and unaware state, the patient *wanted to be kept alive* as long as possible. All family members *disagree* with the patient's previously stated wishes and ask that all life-prolonging treatments, including artificial fluid and nutrition, be stopped. You recommend:

A   Continue routine nursing care but stop all treatments necessary for prolonging life, including artificial fluid and nutrition.

B   Continue fluid and nutrition through artificial means as well as routine nursing care, but do not add any additional procedures or treatments.

C   Continue fluid and nutrition through artificial means as well as routine nursing care, and in addition add the following procedures or treatments if they become necessary for prolonging life (circle as many numbers as apply):

          antibiotics . . . 1
          simple diagnostic tests . . . 2
          invasive diagnostic tests . . . 3
          blood or blood product transfusions . . . 4
          transfer to intensive care unit . . . 5
          dialysis . . . 6
          chemotherapy for cancer . . . 7
          minor surgery . . . 8
          major surgery . . . 9
          mechanical ventilation . . . 10
          cardiopulmonary resuscitation . . . 11
          organ transplantation . . . 12

D   Do everything possible to prolong life, including but not limited to the procedures and treatments listed in C.

E   Other (specify) _____

Please explain or qualify your recommendation:

_____
_____
_____
_____

If all legal and bureaucratic constraints were removed, would your recommendation change?

       YES . . . 1   NO . . . 2

If yes, in what way?

_____
_____
_____
_____

Variation #5: The patient described above left *no oral or written advance directive* of any kind. The family asks that all life-prolonging treatments, including artificial fluid and nutrition, be stopped. You recommend:

A   Continue routine nursing care but stop all treatments necessary for prolonging life, including artificial fluid and nutrition.

B   Continue fluid and nutrition through artificial means as well as routine nursing care, but do not add any additional procedures or treatments.

C   Continue fluid and nutrition through artificial means as well as routine nursing care, and in addition add the following procedures or treatments if they become necessary for prolonging life (circle as many numbers as apply):

antibiotics . . . 1
simple diagnostic tests . . . 2
invasive diagnostic tests . . . 3
blood or blood product transfusions . . . 4
transfer to intensive care unit . . . 5
dialysis . . . 6
chemotherapy for cancer . . . 7
minor surgery . . . 8
major surgery . . . 9
mechanical ventilation . . . 10
cardiopulmonary resuscitation . . . 11
organ transplantation . . . 12

D   Do everything possible to prolong life, including but not limited to the procedures and treatments listed in C.

E   Other (specify) _____

Please explain or qualify your recommendation:

_____

_____

_____

_____

If all legal and bureaucratic constraints were removed, would your recommendation change?

            YES . . . 1   NO . . . 2

If yes, in what way?

_____

_____

_____

_____

Variation #6: The patient described above left *no oral or written advance directive* of any kind. The family asks that "everything possible" be done to prolong life. You recommend:

A   Continue routine nursing care but stop all treatments necessary for prolonging life, including artificial fluid and nutrition.

B   Continue fluid and nutrition through artificial means as well as routine nursing care, but do not add any additional procedures or treatments.

C   Continue fluid and nutrition through artificial means as well as routine nursing care, and in addition add the following procedures or treatments if they become necessary for prolonging life (circle as many numbers as apply):

            antibiotics . . . 1
            simple diagnostic tests . . . 2
            invasive diagnostic tests . . . 3
            blood or blood product transfusions . . . 4
            transfer to intensive care unit . . . 5
            dialysis . . . 6
            chemotherapy for cancer . . . 7
            minor surgery . . . 8
            major surgery . . . 9
            mechanical ventilation . . . 10
            cardiopulmonary resuscitation . . . 11
            organ transplantation . . . 12

D   Do everything possible to prolong life, including but not limited to the procedures and treatments listed in C.

E   Other (specify) _____

Please explain or qualify your recommendation:

_____
_____
_____
_____

If all legal and bureaucratic constraints were removed, would your recommendation change?

        YES . . . 1   NO . . . 2

If yes, in what way?

_____
_____
_____
_____

Variation #7: The patient described above left *no oral or written advance directive* of any kind. There are no known family members or friends. You recommend:

A   Continue routine nursing care but stop all treatments necessary for prolonging life, including artificial fluid and nutrition.

B   Continue fluid and nutrition through artificial means as well as routine nursing care, but do not add any additional procedures or treatments.

C   Continue fluid and nutrition through artificial means as well as routine nursing care, and in addition add the following procedures or treatments if they become necessary for prolonging life (circle as many numbers as apply):

     antibiotics . . . 1
     simple diagnostic tests . . . 2
     invasive diagnostic tests . . . 3
     blood or blood product transfusions . . . 4
     transfer to intensive care unit . . . 5
     dialysis . . . 6
     chemotherapy for cancer . . . 7
     minor surgery . . . 8
     major surgery . . . 9
     mechanical ventilation . . . 10
     cardiopulmonary resuscitation . . . 11
     organ transplantation . . . 12

D   Do everything possible to prolong life, including but not limited to the procedures and treatments listed in C.

E   Other (specify) _____

Please explain or qualify your recommendation:

_____

_____

_____

_____

If all legal and bureaucratic constraints were removed, would your recommendation change?

        YES . . . 1   NO . . . 2

If yes, in what way?

_____

_____

_____

_____

Variation #8: If you were the patient described above, which of the following would you want for yourself?

A   Continue routine nursing care but stop all treatments necessary for prolonging life, including artificial fluid and nutrition.

B   Continue fluid and nutrition through artificial means as well as routine nursing care, but do not add any additional procedures or treatments.

C   Continue fluid and nutrition through artificial means as well as routine nursing care, and in addition add the following procedures or treatments if they become necessary for prolonging life (circle as many numbers as apply):

        antibiotics . . . 1
        simple diagnostic tests . . . 2
        invasive diagnostic tests . . . 3
        blood or blood product transfusions . . . 4
        transfer to intensive care unit . . . 5
        dialysis . . . 6
        chemotherapy for cancer . . . 7
        minor surgery . . . 8
        major surgery . . . 9
        mechanical ventilation . . . 10
        cardiopulmonary resuscitation . . . 11
        organ transplantation . . . 12

D Do everything possible to prolong life, including but not limited to the procedures and treatments listed in C.

E Other (specify) _____

Please explain or qualify your recommendation:

_____

_____

_____

_____

If all legal and bureaucratic constraints were removed, would your recommendation change?

        YES . . . 1   NO . . . 2

If yes, in what way? _____

_____

_____

_____

For each of the following questions, please circle the code number which corresponds to your response or fill in the appropriate blank.

1. In the last three years, have you been a member of an ethics committee?

        YES . . . 1   NO . . . 2

If yes: In what type(s) of organization have you functioned as an ethics committee member? (e.g., university hospital, private hospital, public hospital, HMO, etc.) _____

Approximately how many times in the last three years has your committee made specific recommendations about limiting treatment for particular patient cases?_____

2. In the last three years, have you functioned as an ethics consultant, not including your experience as an ethics committee member?

        YES . . . 1   NO . . . 2

If yes: In what type(s) of organization have you functioned as an ethics consultant? (e.g., university hospital, private hospital, public hospital, HMO, etc.)_

_____

In your experience as an ethics consultant, approximately how many times in the last three years have you made specific recommendations about limiting treatment for particular patient cases?_____

3. Please describe your professional background (e.g., nurse, philosopher, literature professor, etc.) _____

   _____

4. Please list your academic and professional degrees

   _____

5. Sex   M . . . 1   F . . . 2

6. Age   < 30 . . . 1   30-39 . . . 2   40-49 . . . 3   50-59 . . . 4   > 60 . . . 5

7. Religion   Catholic . . . 1
                     Protestant . . . 2
                     Jewish . . . 3
                     Agnostic . . . 4
                     No belief . . . 5
                     Other . . . 6 (specify)_____

8. How religious do you consider yourself to be?

         VERY . . . 1   SOMEWHAT . . . 2   NOT AT ALL . . . 3

9. Do you have a written advance directive which expresses your personal wishes about continuing or limiting treatment in the event of your own inability to make health care decisions?

         YES . . . 1   NO . . . 2

10. Do you have a written advance directive which designates a particular person or persons to act as your proxy decision-maker in the event of your own inability to make health care decisions?
          YES . . . 1   NO . . . 2

Additional comments are welcome. Thank you again for your time.

SOURCE: From "Ethics consultants' recommendations for life-prolonging treatment of patients in a persistent vegetative state," by E. Fox and C. Stocking, 1993, *Journal of the American Medical Association, 270,* pp. 2578-2582. Reprinted with permission.

NOTE: This instrument was developed while Dr. Fox was a faculty member at the MacLean Center for Clinical Medical Ethics at the University of Chicago.

RATIONING HEALTH CARE RESOURCES: SOME CONSIDERED MORAL JUDGMENTS

Developed by Larry W. Foster and
Linda J. McLellan from original work by Leonard Fleck

INSTRUMENT DEVELOPMENT, ADMINISTRATION, AND SCORING

Allocation of health care resources is especially contentious during the current effort to control costs by further rationing services. Allocation decisions are of concern to health professionals who may believe that such policy runs counter to the basic moral tenets of their professions. Understanding similarities and differences in beliefs between professional subgroups about allocation may be important in promoting collaboration and moral discourse to improve patient care.

Because much of the rationing in the United States is hidden and not openly labeled as such (Foster & McLellan, 1997), the items for this instrument were originally developed by Leonard Fleck (1991) as moral judgments to be used in resource allocation for the terminally ill. Respondents are asked to indicate the strength of their convictions for each item on a Likert-type scale (ranging from 1 = strongly disagree to 4 = strongly agree).

PSYCHOMETRIC PROPERTIES

The instrument was administered to 45 social workers, 300 registered nurses working in a medical surgical setting, and 221 physicians in one teaching hospital. Items were derived from work on justice and rationing and are believed to be representative of "ethical cutpoints" in the rationing debate (Fleck, 1991). This study represents one philosopher's distillation of considered moral judgments; no further assessment of content validity could be located.

SUMMARY AND CRITIQUE

The question about personal ADs was included because having one presumes serious consideration of limit setting in end-of-life decisions (Foster & McLellan, 1997). This assumption should be tested. Other validity work needs to be done to characterize the constructs measured. No evidence of reliability testing could be located. The emphasis in work to date has been on describing different philosophical positions by profession. Social workers and physicians expressed more utilitarian beliefs and nurses more egalitarian beliefs in the rationing statements.

Although little information is currently available about the psychometric characteristics of this instrument, Foster (1998) is pursuing this work. The instrument does focus on issues not elsewhere addressed—ones that are very important in the ethical basis for the development of public policy.

REFERENCES

Fleck, L. M. (1991). Just caring: Justice, resource allocation, and the terminally ill. *Ethics-In-Formation, 3*(4&5), 5-7.

Foster, L. W. (1998). Personal communication.

Foster, L. W., & McLellan, L. J. (1997). Moral judgments in the rationing of health care resources: A comparative study of clinical health professionals. *Social Work in Health Care, 25*(4), 13-36.

Instrument 11.2

Rationing Health Care Resources: Some Considered Moral Judgments

S1. No one has an unlimited right to health care

S2. No one has a moral claim to futile or virtually futile health care resources

S3. The social/economic worth of individuals is not a morally relevant consideration in determining fair access to health care resources

S4. Those who have lived out a natural life span have less of a claim to expensive life-prolonging medical resources than those who hope to achieve such a life span

S5. Any rationing proposal/principle that targets the elderly must be coupled with equally effective proposals/principles that reduce the wasteful use of health resources by the non-elderly

S6. No one has a moral claim to merely marginal health benefits especially when there are more urgent unmet health needs in society

S7. The magnitude of a likely benefit from a specific health intervention relative to cost is a morally legitimate consideration in establishing limits and rationing processes

S8. All rationing policy decisions ought to be a product of public, visible decision-making processes

S9. Those who have lost the capacity to have a self, that is, the capacity to have meaningful relations with others, the capacity to connect their past with projects for the future and the capacity to be a center of experience, no longer have just claims to expensive life-prolonging medical resources

S10. No new technologies should be developed or applied to the old that are likely to produce only chronic illness and a short life, to increase the present burden of chronic illness, or to extend the lives of the elderly but offer no significant improvement in their quality of life

S11. A reasonable moral criterion for assessing the relative priority of competing health needs would be the degree to which a specific health intervention protects or restores effective equality of opportunity

S12. It is morally legitimate to give greater priority to funding those health interventions that are likely to forestall death or restore health/function for the relatively younger members of society

S13. Rationing decisions are more likely to be just if they are decisions that are self-imposed rather than being imposed by some (healthy individuals) on others (sick and vulnerable individuals)

S14. No one has a moral claim to non-costworthy health care–or the sort of care that would not be purchased by a reasonable prudent purchaser with a limited budget

S15. Physicians are not morally obligated to do everything medically possible on behalf of their patients because it will often be the case that patients will have no just claim to those resources; or else, they may have a claim, but there may be other patients who have a stronger claim to that same resource

S16. Physicians have no moral right to make unlimited demands upon public resources, or hospital resources, or insurance resources on be-half of their patients, especially when the making of those demands results in making those who are already least well off so far as health is concerned even worse off

S17. Individual patients do have a strong moral right to use their purely private resources in terminal circumstances to purchase what most people would judge to be non-costworthy health care. But they may not use these resources to purchase health goods that are scarce in an absolute sense

S18. Physicians cannot be absolutely uncompromised advocates of a present patient's interests because every physician has other patients (as do health professionals) who make just claims of their time and skills

SOURCE: From "Moral judgments in the rationing of health care resources: A comparative study of clinical health professionals," by L. W. Foster and L. J. McLellan, 1997, Social Work in Health Care, 25(4), pp. 13-36. Adapted with permission from Fleck, L. (1991). Just Caring: Justice, Resource Alloca-tion, and the Terminally Ill, Ethics-In-Formation, 3(4 & 5), pp. 6-7.

12

Summary

Chapter 1 outlined the usefulness of measurement instruments in clinical ethics and the psychometric standards against which they are generally evaluated. After a short review of these standards, this chapter summarizes how the instruments included in the book meet these standards, the needs of the field, and cautions on their use.

Psychometric analysis offers the opportunity to improve the quality of decisions made on the basis of abstract and subjective phenomena such as informed consent or patient preferences. Validity describes the range of interpretations that can appropriately be placed on a measurement score and frequently uses theory to help interpret results. Low levels of reliability (reproducibility across time or raters, or internal consistency) can limit validity. The most important elements of reliability and validity differ by the purpose of the measurements. In prediction of outcomes, test-retest reliability is crucial. Evaluative instruments (those designed to measure longitudinal change over time) must detect clinically important change even if those changes are small (Guyatt, Deyo, Charlson, Levine, & Alba, 1989).

INSTRUMENTS

As a group, the instruments reviewed in this book measure the processes, not outcomes, of ethical decision making and frequently in constructed rather than real situations. The table in the Appendix shows that only a few currently have fully developed scoring systems and well-developed data about validity and reliability. In most instances, reliability does not reach the level outlined in Chapter 1 as necessary for important decisions about individual patients, which is what many of the instruments are designed to do. A very few—even those first developed more than a decade ago—have been used by multiple authors, thereby accumulating evidence of the instrument's measurement characteristics with a range of populations and settings. A common definition of major constructs is unusual, and few instruments are theory based. Many instruments use vignettes extensively with little information about the predictive validity of the scores derived for real clinical situations. The sensitivity of most instruments to intervention has also not been determined.

The consequences of the use of these instruments are virtually unstudied. Thus, from a psychometric viewpoint, this set of instruments is still very young. About two thirds were developed to study or be used with patients; the remaining are geared for application with providers. Many areas of importance to ethicists, patients, and providers are not included in this set of retrieved instruments. Whether measurement instruments exist in these areas is not known with certainty. Examples of constructs for which instruments could not be found include voluntariness for informed consent and most issues related to justice. There are also very few instruments that address ethical issues in health care institutions or communities. The assumption that the individual is the unit of measurement, analysis, and modification is the norm. This may have the unfortunate inadvertent effect of reinforcing the notion that individuals should be the sources of change. Instruments for children could not be located. Those representing particular theoretical perspectives such as feminist or communitarian also could not be found.

In the area of consent, as well as in other areas, there are also no widely accepted, empirically established criteria for determining the quality of the participant's decision-making process or reasonableness of the participant's choice (Tymchuk, 1997), and there are no normative data for what a reasonable person understands in various consent situations. This is particularly problematic because there is substantial evidence suggesting that reasonable people understand little of their research participation or treatment, and those with less-than-average intellectual ability understand the least.

As with many other subject matter areas, this set of measurement instruments was developed primarily with white, middle-class people. Their usefulness with individuals from other cultures is largely unknown. Indeed, some people find the whole notion of "tests" foreign to their thinking, and highly verbal-oriented tests may be problematic for those with limited literacy levels. Although it is clearly relevant, very little work has been done on the social or individual effects of use of these scales, including the potential for test bias with various populations. Detection of bias requires analysis of group by item interactions and evaluating the ability of tests to predict important outcomes for different groups.

INSTRUMENT USE

Some general maxims about instrument use apply. A single test score is by itself only one piece of data for a decision. Instruments should be used only if culturally appropriate interventions are available to help clients. Although not completely accurate, instruments with good measurement characteristics may be the best and fairest methods available to provide information for making decisions. They offer a sample of behavior acquired under standardized conditions with established rules for scoring to obtain quantitative information. Although not an exhaustive measure of all possible behaviors, the best among them should be helpful with potential problems of high variability among examiners, and of having sampled sufficient situations to be generalizable to others.

The social consequences of widespread use of measurement instruments in clinical and research ethics depends on many factors: on the psychometric quality of the tools, the implicit and explicit performance standards inherent in the interpretation and use of scores, how results are used in decisions, and the degree to which the values, ideologies, and theories on which the instruments are based are understood. The use of measurement instruments should stimulate debate and consensus building in the field about these issues. The consequences of their use with all societal groups should be monitored.

In summary, the collection and examination of work on measurement instruments in clinical ethics show robust beginning development and identify areas in which continued work is necessary.

REFERENCES

Guyatt, G. H., Deyo, R. A., Charlson, M., Levine, M. N., & Alba, M. (1989). Responsiveness and validity in health status measurement: A clarification. *Journal of Clinical Epidemiology, 42,* 403-408.

Tymchuk, A. J. (1997). Informing for consent: Concepts and methods. *Canadian Psychology, 38*(2), 55-75.

Instrument A.1

Concept Measured First Author Name	Purports to Measure	Purpose of Measurement	Scoring Guide	Validity		Sensitivity to Interventions	Reliability	
				Content	Construct		Int. Const.	Other*
PT PREFERENCE								
Ende The Autonomy Preference Index (API)	General pt. attitudes toward autonomy	Support shared decision making	Y	Y	Y	N	.82	.84, .83
Cassileth Information Styles Questionnaire (ISQ)	Cancer pts' attitudes toward information and participation in medical decisions		INC	N	N	N	N	N
Thompson Decision Involvement Questionnaire (DIQ)	Desire for input into situations not requiring medical expertise	Delineating boundary in which pts. feel competent to be more autonomous	Y	N	Y	N	.87	N
Danis Desire for Length of Benefit Scale (DLBS) Desire for Probable Benefit Scale (DPBS)	Desire for life-sustaining treatment		Y	?	Y	N	.91, .88	N
Beland Life Support Preference Questionnaire (LSPQ)	Life support preferences	Educate pts. re life support choices	Y	Y	Y	N	N	.73

Concept Measured First Author Name	Purports to Measure	Purpose of Meaurement	Scoring Guide	Validity			Reliability	
				Content	Construct	Sensitivity to Interventions	Int. Const.	Other*
Schonwetter Cardiopulmonary Resuscitation Preference Scale (CPR Pref)	CPR preferences	Pt. informed choice re CPR	Y	N	Y	Y	N	.87
Cohen-Mansfield Preference of Life-Sustaining Treatment Questionnaire (PLSTQ)	Preference for life-sustaining treatments		Y	Y	N	N	N	.81
PT COMPREHENSION								
Krynski Pre-Vignette Knowledge Test Post-Vignette Comprehension Test	Knowledge of enteral feeding	For AD planning	Y	Y	Y	Y	N	N
Lerman Knowledge About Breast Cancer Genetics and BRCA1 Testing Perceptions of the Benefits, Limitations and Risk of BRCA1 Testing	Knowledge re breast cancer genetics and BRCA1 testing and perceptions of benefits, limitations, and risks	Consent for testing	Y	N	Y	Y	Knowledge .74 Perception .83	N

Concept Measured First Author Name	Purports to Measure	Purpose of Measurement	Scoring Guide	Validity		Sensitivity to Interventions	Reliability	
				Content	Construct		Int. Const.	Other*
Elit Decision Board (DB) and Comprehension Questionnaire (CQ)	Understand treatment options for ovarian cancer	Develop treatment preference	Y	Y	Y	Y	N	N
Miller Deaconess Informed Consent Comprehension Test (DICCT)	Consent comprehension for drug trials	Informed choice	Y	Y	?	N	N	.84
DECISIONAL CAPACITY								
Molloy Standardized Mini-Mental State Examination (SMMSE)	Capacity to complete AD and to consent to treatment	Screening test for clinical trials and as outcome measure	Y	N	N	Y	N	.90 interrater .92 intrarater
ADVANCE DIRECTIVES								
Kielstein Values Assessment and Directives Form (VAD)	Story-based values assessment		N	N	N	N	N	N
Doukas Values History (VH)	Values history and AD based on those values		Partial	Y	Y	N	.66-.69	N
Kohut Advance Directive-HIV Questionnaire (AD-HIV)	Pt. preferences for life-sustaining treatment in HIV		Y	Y	N	N	N	N

Concept Measured First Author Name	Purports to Measure	Purpose of Measurement	Scoring Guide	Validity			Reliability	
				Content	Construct	Sensitivity to Interventions	Int. Const.	Other*
Emanuel The Medical Directive (MD)	Advance directive with multiple scenarios and treatment decisions		N	Y	Y	N	.93 public .97 MDs	72%
Singer Advance Directive Acceptability Questionnaire (ADAQ)	Acceptability of AD forms		Y	Y	N	N	.93	N
Heffner Advance Directives Questionnaire (ADQ)	End-of-life decision making for pts. with chronic obstructive lung disease		Inc	N	Y	Y	N	90%
Stoeckle End-of-Life Questionnaire (EOLCDQ II)	Provider compliance with PSDA			Y	Y	N	.85	N
WITHDRAWAL OF LIFE SUPPORT								
Cook Withdrawal of Life Support in Critically Ill Patients	Values of health care workers re withdrawal of life support		N	Y	N	N	N	.68-.96
Christakis Willingness to Withdraw Life Support (WWLS)	Physician likelihood of withdrawing life support	Document bias to involved physicians	Y	Y	Y	N	.79	N

Concept Measured First Author Name	Purports to Measure	Purpose of Meaurement	Scoring Guide	Validity		Sensitivity to Interventions	Reliability	
				Content	Construct		Int. Const.	Other*
AGGRESSIVENESS OF CARE								
Baggs Decisions about Aggressiveness of Care (DAC) Decisions about Aggressiveness of Care for Specific Patients (DAC[SP])	Providers' views about how aggressively to treat ICU pts.		N	Y	N	N	.74	.73
Shelley Aggressiveness of Nursing Care Scale (ANCS)	Beliefs regarding aggressiveness of nursing care		Y	Y	N	N	.81	N
Raines Level of Management in Neonatal Clinical Situations	Providers' views about aggressiveness of care and relevant information.		Y	Y	Y	N	.62-.89	N
MORAL SENSITIVITY								
Lutzen Moral Sensitivity Questionnaire (MSQ)	Experience of moral decision making in psychiatric practice	Identify differences in ethical problems in a practice team	Y	Y	Y	N	.73, .78 Nurses .64 Psychiatrists	N
ETHICS ENVIRONMENT								
McDaniel Ethics Environment Questionnaire (EEQ)	Ethics work environment	Particularly focused on nurses	Y	Y	Y	Y	.93	.88

Concept Measured First Author Name	Purports to Measure	Purpose of Meaurement	Scoring Guide	Validity		Sensitivity to Interventions	Reliability	
				Content	Construct		Int. Const.	Other*
Olson Hospital Ethical Climate Survey (HECS)	Hospital ethical	Particularly focused on nurses	Y	Y	Y	N	.91	N
RECIPIENT SELECTION								
Corley Criteria for Selection of Transplant Recipient Scale (CSTR)	Criteria for selection of organ transplant recipients		Y	Y	N	N	N	.85
GENERAL ISSUES FOR HEALTH PROFESSIONALS								
Fox Ethics Consultant's Recommendations (ECR)	Consistency of ethics consultants' recommendations		Y	N	N	N	N	N
Foster Rationing Health Care Resources: Some Considered Moral Judgments	Moral judgments about rationing health care resources		Y	N	N	N	N	N
*Test-Retest	AD = Advance directive							
Inc = Incomplete	Int. Consist = Internal Consistency							

Y = Yes, N = No, Inc = Incomplete, ? = Not Clear

Index

About the Author

Barbara Klug Redman, Ph.D., is Dean and Professor at Wayne State University College of Nursing. She received her master's and Ph.D. degrees from the University of Minnesota, was a postdoctoral fellow at the Johns Hopkins University School of Public Health, a Visiting Fellow at the Kennedy Institute of Ethics at Georgetown University, and a Fellow in Medical Ethics at Harvard Medical School. She previously served as Executive Director of the American Association of Colleges of Nursing and later as Executive Director of the American Nurses Association and has held faculty and administrative appointments at the University of Washington, the University of Minnesota, the University of Colorado, the University of Connecticut, and the Johns Hopkins University. Dr. Redman holds honorary doctorates from Georgetown University and the University of Colorado and an Outstanding Achievement Award from the University of Minnesota Board of Regents.